Jazz Dance Today

Jazz Dance Today

Lorraine Person Kriegel

Kimberly Chandler-Vaccaro

Series Editor for West's Physical Activities Series

Robert J. O'Connor, Ed.D.
Los Angeles Pierce College

West Publishing Company
Minneapolis/St. Paul   New York   Los Angeles   San Francisco

Composition: Patti Zeman, Moorpark, CA
Photography: Lev Nisnevitch
Computer Illustration/Production: Miyake Illustration & Design

WEST'S COMMITMENT TO THE ENVIRONMENT
In 1906, West Publishing Company began recycling materials left over from the
production of books. This began a tradition of efficient and responsible use of
resources. Today, up to 95 percent of our legal books and 70 percent of our
college and school texts are printed on recycled, acid-free stock. West also
recycles nearly 22 million pounds of scrap paper annually—the equivalent of
181,717 trees. Since the 1960s, West has devised ways to capture and recycle
waste inks, solvents, oils, and vapors created in the printing process. We also
recycle plastics of all kinds, wood, glass, corrugated cardboard, and batteries,
and have eliminated the use of Styrofoam book packaging. We at West are
proud of the longevity and the scope of our commitment to the environment.

Production, Prepress, Printing and Binding by West Publishing Company

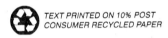 *TEXT PRINTED ON 10% POST
CONSUMER RECYCLED PAPER*

Copyright © 1994   By WEST PUBLISHING COMPANY
                          610 Opperman Drive
                          P.O. Box 64526
                          St. Paul, MN 55164-0526

Printed in the United States of America

8 7 6 5 4

Library of Congress Cataloging-in-Publication Data

Kriegel, Lorraine Person.
    Jazz dance today / Lorraine Person Kriegel, Kimberly Chandler-Vaccaro.
    p. cm.—(West's physical activities series)
    Includes index.
    ISBN 0-314-02717-3
    1. Jazz dance.   I. Chandler-Vaccaro, Kimberly.   II. Title.
GV1784.K75   1994   93-41158
793.3—dc20   ∞   CIP

Dedication

With thanks to my mother, Elise Person, for her gift of dance. With hope that my daughter, Jessica Kriegel, finds a passion as joyful, if different. With gratitude for the support and love of Hubert.

Lorraine Person Kriegel

To Wayne, with love

Kimberly Chandler-Vaccaro

Table of Contents

Chapter 4	**Basic Nutrition and Cardiorespiratory Conditioning**	**43**

Chapter 5	**Supplemental Strength Training for the Dancer**	**53**

Chapter 6	**Supplemental Flexibility Training for the Dancer**	**63**

Chapter 7	**Discipline and Training Schedules**	**69**

Preface

Jazz dance is a nonverbal art form traditionally passed from teacher to student in a physical way. In preparing a book about jazz dance—in effect making the nonverbal verbal—we have tried to integrate written information from dance theorists, historians, and kinesiologists with dance information from teachers, choreographers, producers, and dancers. Our goal was to present an accurate picture of jazz dance today in the context of its tradition supported by the latest in dance science research. Our purpose in bringing this information together was to supplement the more emotional and immediate experience of jazz dance classes with a conceptual structure that will enrich the studio experience for the students.

This past decade has seen a surge in the theoretical information written on dance. Dance as an art form is being researched, analyzed, and studied in terms of both history and creative processes, while dance kinesiology, the science of dance movement, is a rapidly expanding field. Each area offers its own insights into the dance arena, and dancers today have the advantage of applying this information to their daily training.

Jazz Dance Today includes the findings of current research. It is an organizational framework based on the principles of dance fitness, allowing the student and teacher to concentrate on the art. On the surface, it will appear not unlike a traditional class, yet the exercises have been ordered and conceived to provide a balance of strength and flexibility, endurance conditioning, and neuromuscular coordination. The class is broken down into elements, each defined by current information on dance kinesiology.

Consideration is given to the idea of dance as an entity in itself and as a mind-body-soul application. We believe that intention, expressiveness, motivation, performance quality, musicality, and communication within the art of dance are foremost. Our framework allows students to work on these attributes knowing they are attending to physical wellness. In an attempt to bypass some of the injuries that have plagued dancers for so long, the framework is a strategy that emphasizes student safety in a comprehensive dance experience. *Jazz Dance Today* provides a visual tool to examine a dancer's training. It is meant as a practical guide that can free class time for dancing.

Jazz dance is a freedom-loving, movement-loving tradition. Each young jazz dancer who receives this gift of expression is free to play with it and shape it to his or her own world view. Therefore, jazz dance today is not jazz dance yesterday or jazz dance tomorrow.

We would like to thank the dance masters who gave so willingly of their time and expertise and our teachers and mentors who gave us the passion for jazz dance.

Judith Alter

Brenda Bufalino

Danny Buraczeski

Patrick Campbell

Rene Cebalos

Russell Clark

Gary Cowan

Rhett Dennis

Judith Gantz

Rob Gibson

Hama

Frank Hatchett

Luigi

Ben Lokey

Matt Mattox

Albert Murray

Molly Molloy

Max Roach

Francis Roach

Billy Siegenfeld

Lynn Simonson

David Storey

Susan Stoman

In addition, we were very fortunate to have the following dance educators review several versions of this manuscript and offer constructive and valuable advice: Jaime Aiken, Teresa Benzwie, Jo Dierdorff, Martha Dowell, Michael J. Eger, Dorothy Garant, Alfred Hansen, Joan Hays, Barbara Lappano, Cindy Lewis, Nina Lucas, Tony Marich, Wanda Martin-McGill, Angela Schnee, and Debora Tell.

Our editors at West Publishing were patient beyond reason with our fledgling attempts to capture jazz dance in a readable and accessible form. Theresa O'Dell granted us tenacious assistance, and, after we had a tentative manuscript, Beth Kennedy and Allen Gooch were endlessly meticulous and supportive.

Thank you for Princeton Book Company's permission to reprint from Doris Humphrey's The Art of Making Dances.

Several friends helped, as friends do, with opinions, advice, emotional support, and typing skills: Todd Murey, Laura McMuray, and Isadora Kriegel.

Finally, thank you to our families who gave up so much so that we could pursue this undertaking: Hubert and Jessica Kriegel, and Wayne and Chandler Vaccaro.

Lorraine Person Kriegel
Kimberly Chandler-Vaccaro

The Series Editor for West's Physical Activities Series

The Series Editor for West's Physical Activities Series is Dr. Bob O'Connor, Los Angeles Pierce College. Dr. O'Connor received his B.S. and M.S. degrees in physical education from UCLA and his doctorate from U.S.C. His 30-year teaching experience includes instruction in physical education courses of tennis, weight training, volleyball, badminton, swimming and various team sports, as well as classes in teaching methods. He brings to the Series a wide range of college coaching experience in areas of swimming, tennis, water polo, and football. Internationally, Dr. O'Connor has been an advisor to several Olympic programs in weight training and swimming. He was among the first to popularize strength training for all athletic events. Dr. O'Connor has written extensively in the fields of physical education and health and is a dedicated advocate of physical education TODAY.

Books in West's Physical Activities Series

Aerobics Today by Carole Casten and Peg Jordan
Aqua Aerobics Today by Carole Casten
Badminton Today by Tariq Wadood and Karlyne Tan
Jazz Dance Today by Lorraine Person Kriegel and Kimberly Chandler-Vaccaro
Golf Today by J.C. Snead and John Johnson
Racquetball Today by Lynn Adams and Erwin Goldbloom
Swimming and Aquatics Today by Ron Ballatore and William Miller
Tennis Today by Glenn Bassett and William Otta
Volleyball Today by Marv Dunphy and Rod Wilde
Weight Training Today by Robert O'Connor, Jerry Simmons, and J. Patrick O'Shea

Introduction

Jazz Dance Today, by Luigi

Before he became a teacher, Luigi was already a successful dancer. He worked for many years dancing and choreographing in nightclubs, television, films, and the theater. When he arrived on Broadway, it wasn't long before other professional dancers, recognizing the purity of his dancing style, asked him to teach. Each had a special request: "Teach me how to jump like that!" "Why are your turns so secure?" "Where is your balance coming from?" What all his students eventually learned was that his technique was not just a combination of separate skills but a unified art that came from within and started at the very beginning. He went on to become the most influential jazz dancer in the world, with honors flowing in from United States presidents, state governors, and mayors around the world. On March 21, 1990, Luigi Day was proclaimed in New York City.

His success in itself is remarkable, but it becomes all the more inspiring when one learns that Luigi developed his technique after waking up from an extended coma, unable to walk or see, paralyzed on one side of his body—the result of a car accident when he was twenty-one. His goal as he left the hospital was not just to walk again but to dance; his method was, simply, to start dancing. He fell a lot . . . and he picked himself up and tried not to fall again. This was the beginning of the Luigi Technique. He learned to dance from the very beginning—from the desire—and everything developed from that. It required more than dedication and discipline, it required spiritual strength as well. As he says himself, "First I learned to love, then I learned to dance."

Through his school in New York have passed many dance greats and many leading actors and actresses. They came to learn how to feel, how to focus, how to dance, how to perform. Many have gone on to teach the "Luigi Technique" in studios all over the world. In today's professional jazz dance world, so pervasive is his influence that it is safe to say that there's a part of Luigi in every jazz dance class and in every jazz dancer. He currently teaches in New York and inspires yet another generation of jazz dance artists to learn to love . . . and to dance.

Luigi:

What is *Jazz Dance Today?* The authors of this book have asked that question and tried to answer it in what follows, and I've been asked to write an introduction. Actually, jazz dance today is no different than it was when I started teaching forty-four years ago. There have been changes in music and style perhaps, and there have been lots of fads. But jazz, the real jazz—the thing that makes jazz *jazz*—is no different now than it was then. Jazz, itself, is a feeling—an honest, personal feeling—inspired by soulful music. Jazz *dance* is moving with that feeling through a safe and effective technique. I want the students in my classes to learn to *feel* as they move through my exercises and choreography. I want them to look inside themselves and discover who they are. I want them to learn control, balance, extensions, and focus by finding the source inside themselves. The source of jazz is inside. This is what I have tried to teach my students since the very beginning and what I hope will be my legacy.

When I dance, I'm telling you all about myself. I don't want my students to dance like I do; I don't want them to dance what I feel—my feeling is *my* feeling—I want them to dance *their* feelings. Not all dancers do that; a lot hold back. Maybe they hold back because they don't want others to see who they are. Maybe they're afraid that a part of them—a part that they don't like—will show. If a person has no feeling, it's because he has never looked inside himself, he has not found himself. It's there, but if he hasn't found it, then he's not a jazz dancer.

As a teacher, that's my goal: to get to the feeling inside. My first bit of advice: Don't think of what you have done or will be doing; think only in the *now*. You are what you are right now.

Jazz dancing is also technique, skill, craft. I developed the Luigi Technique to help dancers learn about their bodies—how to control it, how to gain strength and line. The Luigi Technique is an integration of the body into dance. I don't believe in isolations; I believe in the body becoming whole and balanced. Everything should contribute to the feeling, and everything comes from the feeling.

Part of moving from the inside means that you dance within the limits of your own body, and you do only what you feel. Jazz dance is such a personal thing that it's just not necessary to go beyond the limits of what you feel. Never force an extension or a back arch. Never lose control. Nothing should hurt. Technique is like tuning an instrument: Learn to tune your body just right, so that when you go to play it, it's beautiful. The beauty of dancing is the control of it.

Again, jazz cannot be found in a pose, or a leap, or a bump, or a grind. It's not a series of "jazz steps." Jazz must always be an honest expression of a musical soul. They say that when you die, your soul leaves your body. Don't wait for your soul to die. Look into your living soul and dance with it . . . simply, honestly, truly.

So many of my students have gone on to teach, choreograph, act, dance, and create all over the world. I want to thank them for carrying on my work and for spreading the joy of jazz dance to so many people, and I want to encourage them to continue . . . never stop moving.

New York
July, 1993

CHAPTER 1

Preparing for the Jazz Dance Class

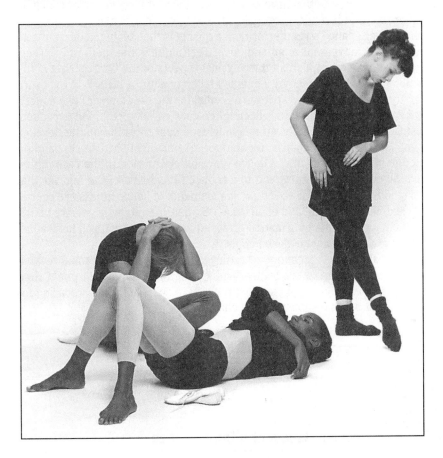

Outline

Knowing What You Want to Achieve and How to Achieve It

The purpose of the jazz dance class today is to train the dancer in a variety of areas: performance qualities and style,[1] dance technique,[2] neuromuscular coordination, musicality, movement memory, and dance fitness.[3] These goals are reached through classes that have evolved over the past forty years[4] and include a warm-up, technique work, vocabulary development, performance, and choreography in a jazz dance style. Performance quality is the ability to communicate the meaning of movement to an audience. Technique is the method or procedure one uses to accomplish all the physical aspects of the dance. Style is the distinction given to the dance by a character, personality, or school. "[5] Exposure to a variety of techniques and styles is essential for the development of a dancer.

Jazz dance classes today are reflecting the current value put upon exceptional physical prowess and ability with an increased concentration on the development of sophisticated dance technique. Simultaneously, an expanding knowledge of biomechanics and dance kinesiology[6] has led to the recognition that overall dance fitness may lead to a reduced incidence of the injuries that have plagued the dancer for so long. (The elements of dance fitness are coordination, flexibility, strength, and endurance.) By determining why you are taking a class then applying the information provided in this book, you will have a better chance of achieving your dance goals.

These goals, however, cannot be achieved without taking personal responsibility for your own progress. Dancers must first understand their goals, then come to class mentally and physically prepared to achieve them. Preparing for a jazz dance class is the subject of this chapter.

Checklist: Goals of a Dance Class

- Develop *performance qualities and style* and the ability to communicate the meaning of movement.
- Develop *dance technique* (alignment, rotation, centering, and transference of weight).
- Develop *neuromuscular coordination* (precise control of placement and movement of all body parts in relation to the choreography).
- Enhance *rhythm and musicality* (how the movement relates to the music).
- Improve *movement memory* (the ability to pick up movements faster, remember them longer, and move in unison with others in the class).
- Improve *dance fitness* (strength, flexibility, coordination, and endurance).
- Develop the stamina and concentration to match the requirements of daily rehearsals and performances.

What to Wear and Why

Dance apparel in the eighties became fashionable as everyday attire. Leg warmers, leotards, and other accoutrements of the dance aesthetic were visible in the general population's clothing. In the nineties, jazz dance wear and sportswear include an array of brightly colored, skintight tops and shorts. Lycra, cotton, and spandex materials are abundant. In choosing clothes for class, however, let reason instead of fashion dictate what you wear and remember simple is often best. Being properly outfitted will enable you to concentrate on the important aspects of class, relieve your mind of unnecessary worries, and ensure your comfort and your safety in some instances.

Close-fitting yet flexible clothes are really a necessity of serious dance training. In dance, every motion is a communication to the audience and the dancer needs to be acutely aware of how every inch of his or her body appears. Conforming clothes allow the dancer to see his or her entire body and allow the teacher to observe and make the appropriate technical corrections. Every curve of the back and bend of the leg is a part of the expressiveness of the art form, and every movement a part of the technique. For these reasons, simple leotards and tights are best. Cotton or cotton blends are the choice fabrics as they allow your skin to breathe and absorb moisture from perspiration. It is especially important for women who dance intensely and often to wear articles that have crotches with cotton linings. This will reduce the incidence of yeast and urinary infections due to moisture.

The past two decades have seen an increase in the athleticism and acrobatics of jazz dancing. This makes it important to cover the legs completely to the ankle. Though shorts may afford more comfort in warm weather, they leave the knees and shins unprotected and possibly exposed to floor burns and bruises. Bearing weight on body parts other than the feet is not uncommon, and this should be taken into consideration before dressing. The back should also be covered, with zippers only on the parts of clothing that are not going to bear weight.

Many dancers avow the practice of wearing leg warmers to keep the ankles warm, soft and pliable. To do much good the material needs to cover the large muscles of the lower leg as well as the ankles. Bulky, extra material surrounding the ankle may impede the instructor's ability to monitor the dancer's technique, however, so it is best to ask each individual teacher his or her preference.

There are many styles of jazz shoes and boots on the market. Though also made of soft leather, the jazz shoe differs from a ballet slipper. The shoe usually laces up the front and sports a small, flat heel. The soles of the shoe are the most important part. They need to be appropriate to the surface of the dance floor. For instance, a slippery wooden floor may accommodate rubber soles, while a floor of marley (a rubberized dance floor) needs leather soles only. Check the floor surface of the studio or studios before you buy shoes if you do not have the luxury of affording two pairs. Wearing footed tights or socks will lengthen the life of your shoes and reduce the chance of athlete's foot by absorbing perspiration. Character shoes (those made of stiffer leather, with larger heels and buckles for women) should be reserved for intermediate and advanced dancers who need to wear them for performances. Beginning dancers should try to master alignment and centering before venturing into shoes that dramatically alter balance and technique.

Understanding the Necessity of Training

There is a contradiction today between the high level of technical training received in class and the apparent abandonment of technique in some current choreography. For example, hip-hop is a recently emerged, popular style of dancing in the music-video medium. It is repetitive and very aerobic but not *technical* in the historical dance sense. Consequently, the rigorous and specialized training of the traditional jazz dance class may seem unnecessary and irrelevant to the young dancer who is used to seeing "street dancing" in so many music videos. Don't be fooled. The flexibility needed for professional dance can only be developed systematically and thoughtfully; stamina and the ability to bear weight on many body parts take intensive strength training, and sufficient coordination is needed for the complexities of choreography. Though it's not evident in every step, conscientious and directed training is necessary to safely achieve the physical prowess, athleticism, and precision necessary for jazz dance.

Terminology

As an art form, ballet has a long, continuous, defined history spanning most of the past four centuries. Jazz dance, on the other hand, with its inception in this century, is relatively new and constantly changing form, steps, and style. Jazz is a more personal art form, based on a unique relationship between the current cultural trends, the performer, choreographer, and the music. This constant, restless inventiveness accounts for both the variety of steps seen in jazz dance classes and the difficulty in attempting to define the exact steps of jazz dance. As much as it uses traditional jazz steps (vernacular jazz dance), jazz also borrows much of the codified French ballet terminology and many of the exercises for its training.[7] Exercises such as *tendu* (tahn-doo'), degagé (day-ga-'jay'), plié (plee-yay'), developpé (dev-el-o-pay'), and grand battement (grahn bot-mahn') have been adapted to the jazz idiom and form part of the basis of jazz dance training. (These exercises are detailed in chapter 3.)

Some familiar, uniquely jazzy moves have survived, however, through the century and have become part of a generally accepted jazz vocabulary. Among them are the jazz contraction, hinge, and kick-ball-change.

Because the stylistic preference of the teacher/choreographer is the main determinant of specific exercises and steps, this vocabulary may or may not appear in your dance class. Over the years, however, the work of some master teachers has greatly influenced what goes on in a jazz class. Teachers such as Luigi, Matt Mattox, and Gus Giordano have designed techniques that perfectly embody their individual jazz styles, and these exercises have found their way into classes across the country and, indeed, the world. It is the integration of current cultural, vernacular dance trends with modern and ballet dance forms that makes jazz, jazz. (Please see chapter 8.)

> "Specific dance steps appear and reappear with surprising regularity over a span of years. Philosophically speaking, American stage dance enjoys both a linear tradition . . . and a tradition of vertical integration in which varied and often irreconcilable forms coexist simultaneously—ballet, modern, concert dance, ballroom, tap, and jazz.

Jazz contraction. See chapter 2 for a complete description of the contraction.

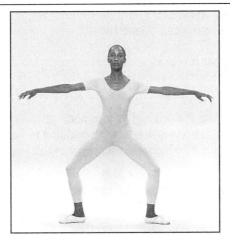 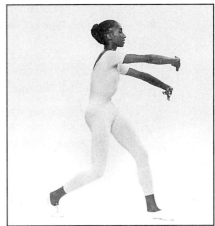

a.   b.

If used in choreography the hinge requires strength in the front of the thighs. In class it is used to develop this strength and is a stylized way to change the level of the pelvis.

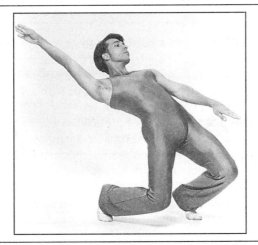

Kick-ball-change is a very common jazz and tap dance step. It has a syncopated rhythm and is often done as a transition or preparatory movement. After a small kick of the lower leg, the weight is shifted briefly from one foot to the other. For example, with the weight on the left foot, kick the right foot on the count of 1. Step onto the right on the count of *and*, and back on the left on the count of 2.

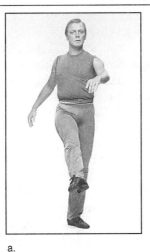 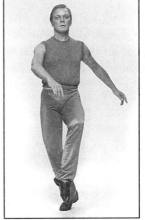 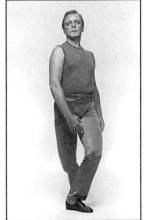

a.   b.   c.

The American show dance embraces them all, often with several types of dance appearing in one show."[8]

"It doesn't matter if you are a classical dancer, a tap dancer, or a modern dancer, the more versatile you can be by knowing all forms of technique, the greater you will be as a specialist."   Matt Mattox[9]

What survives from the original dances performed on street corners and in gin joints where jazz dance was born is the tradition of vernacular dancing, and it remains the standard by which we instantly recognize jazz dancing from other dance forms.

"The vernacular tradition, or the invention of movement, can never be scrapped."[10]

Jazz, with its constant change and inventiveness, as we will continue to investigate throughout this book, *is a living art form.*

Listening to Music in Class

Part of the fun and energy of a jazz class comes from the relationship between the dance and the music. Though some argue that jazz dance must be done exclusively to jazz music, frequently the accompaniment is the most popular and upbeat of the current time.[11] Danceable music with great rhythm contributes much to the atmosphere of the jazz class.

Whatever music is used, it must be treated as an important part of the class. It is not merely background noise nor a catchy metronome but a springboard for inspiration and motivation. All the music's synchronizations and rhythmic qualities should be understood and appreciated. Its melody and drive need to be physically experienced. Constant attention to the music adds greater depth to the student's training. The dance/music relationship is very important. For more on the relationship of music and dance, see chapter 8.

Getting Prepared Mentally

To be mentally ready for class means to have the mind prepared to work with the body at the maximum level of proficiency. Taking a few moments to relax, focus, and coach the mind before class will enable the dancer to be mentally ready to dance and perform. Dancers can profit from recent research done in sports kinesiology to understand the importance of mental preparedness. According to Jean M. Williams in *Applied Sports Psychology*, for peak performance an athlete must be both relaxed and highly focused.[12] In dance, we often speak of this optimum condition as that of being "centered."

"Centered" is a dance term with multiple meanings. Most simply, center refers to the center of the body, or the center of weight. To be centered can mean to have achieved a sense of balance, both physically and emotionally, or may simply imply a good working alignment of the bones and muscles. Dance as an art engages the mind, body, and spirit. In this sense, "to be centered" means to be in a state of appropriate focus and concentration; to be connected to the muscles and bones in a knowing and secure way that results in a free and easy balance; to be aware of the communicative powers of movement; and to be able to express oneself through the dance medium.

Following are two techniques that can help center the dancer and optimize learning.

Psychoneuromuscular Theory[13]

Psychoneuromuscular is the name of the theory that explains how electrical and chemical impulses, similar to those sent from the brain to the muscles during movement, also occur when one merely *imagines* the movement. This means that one can actually practice a movement by imagining it, though the muscle contraction will not be as intense. This activity, also called *imaging*, allows the dancer to mentally and physically rehearse a movement or combination. Since the development of coordination depends on the ability of the brain to send impulses through neural pathways, any rehearsal, physically acted or imaged, will help in the training of the dancer.

There are two types of imaging; internal visualization and external visualization. Internal visualization is imagining the muscles and bones moving from the inside, imagining how they feel in action. External visualization is most like watching television and seeing oneself do a movement.

During the warm-up, visualizing the muscles as being relaxed, soft, and pliable will help one to achieve physical readiness. Imagining the feeling of being concentrated and alert helps the dancer achieve the proper frame of mind for class. Both types of imaging are beneficial in training and help the muscles and mind warmup in the desired fashion. It is very important to imagine yourself doing the movements correctly to ensure a good rehearsal.

As a learning tool, the technique of imaging may be applied to every aspect of your dance training.

Relaxation

There seems to be no end to the research done on the benefits of relaxation in the domains of sports and dance. Relaxation is a pleasurable experience for the central nervous system and very important for the dancer in developing flexibility and balance. (Certain muscles need to be relaxed so that others are able to stretch.) Relaxation is a prerequisite for optimal learning and is profoundly different from fatigue. It can be understood as a feeling of fearlessness, confidence, energy, focus, and calm. By taking a few moments to clear one's mind of unnecessary thoughts, reducing interferences, taking deep and continuous breaths, and consciously telling oneself to relax, the dancer will approach the ideal state for applying the psychoneuromuscular theory. This is something the student can do for himself before the class begins.

In order to be "centered" and ready to get the most out of a dance class, one should be mentally and physically relaxed, focused, and energized. By doing a few simple breathing and imaging exercises, the dancer may be able to achieve this state more rapidly.

Example: Done in Silence

Lying on the back with the knees bent and the feet flat on the floor close to the buttocks, feel the shoulders, the back of the neck, and spine falling gently into the floor. Imagine the sections of the body touching the floor as relaxed and soft. Inhale and exhale fully. Continue to breathe deeply while suggesting to yourself that you are ready to dance. With every breath, tell yourself that you have all the energy and confidence you need to accomplish your goals during class. Imagine your abdominals as strong and able to support your torso. Contract the abdominals and feel the strength in the lower torso and back. Imagine the range of motion in the hips as being full and easy, the length of hamstrings long and loose. Breathe and tell yourself you are operating with the mind, body and emotions in accord. Take a few minutes to set some goals such as keeping the shoulders in line throughout class or listening more intently to the accompaniment. Roll to the side, onto the knees, tuck the toes under the feet, rock back onto the heels and slowly roll up through the spine, visualizing one vertebra at a time unfolding. Keep breathing and engaging the abdominals. Take another deep breath as you come to an energized, well-aligned standing position.

Because we think with our entire being, every change in our emotional and mental state produces a change in our physical state. As we saw in the psychoneuromuscular theory, every thought produces a simultaneous chemical or physical impulse. Any kind of stress or tension can use up energy stored in the body, thus reducing one's strength. It is important to be able to relax in between exercises, rehearsals, and performances.

The mind and body are equal partners in the field of dance; they must be used harmoniously to achieve optimum results. It behooves all dancers to understand the value of imaging and relaxation in their training.

Checklist: Mental Preparation

- Inhale and exhale fully, prompting yourself to be relaxed.
- Free yourself of tension, eliminate any stressful thoughts, and concentrate fully on the class to come.
- Watch the teacher carefully during the demonstrations.
- Use external visualization to imagine yourself doing the exercises as if on TV.
- Imagine how the muscles would *feel* if they were doing the exercise.
- Focus and prepare for a great class!!!

Getting Prepared Physically

"Warm-up" is another dance term with multiple connotations. It implies both a physical and mental readiness for dance, which includes being emotionally and bodily "centered."

In the strict physical application, "warm-up" is the term used to describe the motions that serve to elevate body temperature and improve the circulation of joint and muscular fluids in preparation for the more strenuous exercises that follow. These movements may target a specific area of the body or a muscle group, or they may correspond directly to choreography that will be done full-out later in class. In chapter 3, the "warm-up" includes the first six elements of the class.

The point of the warm-up is to raise the heart rate slowly and increase blood circulation to the muscles so that they become more pliable and responsive. Warm-up exercises should always include full, circular breathing: a conscious, continuous execution of inhalations and exhalations. Breathing should be natural and unexaggerated.[15] An adequate warm-up will increase: the amount of oxygen you are taking in; the aerobic metabolism of the muscles (their ability to use oxygen); and the blood flow in the lungs while diverting some blood flow from the organs and skin to the muscles. Simultaneously, it will increase the nervous system's ability to transmit impulses to contract muscle fibers.

During this time you will check the body to see which muscles are sore or stiff and need attention. You will improve the range of motion of the joints to help prevent subsequent soreness[16] and possibly reduce the frequency of soft-tissue injuries.[17] All this will heighten your ability to become centered or your physical and mental readiness for dance.

Your Personal Warm-up

Since each dancer's body is different, it is important for the dancer to be keenly aware of his or her own physical capabilities and limitations. Being ready to dance full-out is an individual feeling. Therefore, dancers have the responsibility to do any additional necessary movements before class, between exercises, and during any class breaks to ensure a proper warm-up. A good warm-up routine would include several minutes of slow, smooth movements, reaching to the extreme positions. During this time, the dancer can check the body to see which muscles are sore, which need extra care, and what feels good. When this is executed with conscientious mental preparation, the dancer will become more and more in tune to his or her individual needs—a necessary step toward the mastery of the body.

Example:

Imagine yourself standing on the six of a giant clock with the twelve directly above your head. Close your eyes, take two or three deep, full breaths while lengthening the spine gently. Open your eyes. In a slow, meditative fashion, reach with the right arm across the body to the 11:00 position of the clock, then with the left to the 2:00. Next with the right to the 9:00 position, then with the left to the 3:00; again with the right to the 7:00, and with the left to the 4:00. Keep reaching with opposite arms across the body or reach to the same side. Go up to the twelve with both and down to the six. Reach to the extreme points gently, really trying to imagine which muscles are moving and feeling how each does the movement. Clear all other thoughts away. Keep breathing. Visualize relaxed yet energized muscles. Note any

quirks or irregularities in the body. Do movements to stretch or contract any area necessary. Keep breathing; tell yourself you have the
energy you need and the skill to accomplish what is coming next. Be
sure to pay attention to any sore body parts, perhaps massaging
them or doing extra movements for them.

Checklist: Benefits of an Adequate Warm-up

- Increases the amount of oxygen you are taking in and increases the aerobic metabolism of the muscles.
- Increases the blood flow in the lungs and diverts some blood flow from the organs and skin to the muscles.
- Increases the nervous system's ability to transmit impulses and to contract muscle fibers.
- Increases the range of motion in the joints and helps prevent muscle soreness.
- Possibly reduces the frequency of soft-tissue injuries.
- Improves "centering" ability by preparing one mentally and physically to dance.

What's Missing from a Jazz Dance Class

Because of the sheer amount and depth of *technique* training required by today's
jazz dancer, not all dance *fitness* goals can be completely met within the time limits of the traditional jazz dance class. Again, the elements of dance fitness are
strength, flexibility, coordination, and *endurance*. Dance classes involve strength
exercises (pliés, developpés, abdominal work, push-ups, etc.); flexibility work
(stretches, ronds de jambe, isolations, arches, contractions, etc.); and coordination practice (skill development and vocabulary practice). Yet often classes must
be supplemented with additional weight or flexibility training[18] and perhaps indi-
vidualized body therapies[19] to ensure that the dancer is developing in each of
the fitness areas adequately. What is most often missing from class is an
endurance element, or a complete aerobic workout, which helps prepare the
dancer for the high energy demands of the profession. Simply, an aerobic
workout uses oxygen and is a cardiovascular conditioner. To achieve aerobic
conditioning, there must be twelve to thirty minutes of continuous, low-intensity
activity. Dedication of this amount of time is often prohibitive in a 1.5 hour jazz
dance class. The repetition of the longer combinations (forty-five to sixty seconds in length) may be the only aerobic-like activity done during class. In which
case, additional cardiovascular or aerobic workouts may be necessary.[20]

Fit dancers are better dancers and better performers. They have a lower risk
of injury and are more likely to enjoy longer and more rewarding careers. Be
sure to examine your training for all the fitness elements and supplement where

necessary. The elements of the dance class that correspond to those of dance fitness are discussed in chapter 3.

Summary

To fully prepare for the jazz dance class, dancers must take personal responsibility for themselves. They must first understand the purpose and goals of the dance class and come mentally and physically prepared to achieve them. The goals are: to develop a level of *performance quality*, *style*, *dance technique*, and *neuromuscular coordination*; to enhance *musicality*; and to improve *movement memory* and overall *dance fitness*.

To optimize learning, to be centered, and get the most out of class, the dancer needs to be mentally and physically ready. Mental readiness includes relaxing the body and the mind and being able to visualize yourself performing the warm-up correctly and comfortably. The psychoneuromuscular theory is a technique to help the dancer get mentally prepared.

Physical readiness is when the body is prepared to move full-out. Remember to check the body often to ensure that it is properly warmed-up. Pay attention to what feels good and what doesn't as you move slowly and breathe fully.

An adequate warm-up[21] will increase the amount of oxygen you are taking in, the aerobic metabolism of the muscles, and the blood flow in the lungs. It will divert some blood flow from the organs and skin to the muscles. It will raise the heart rate slowly and increase blood circulation to the muscles so that they become more pliable and responsive, increase the nervous system's ability to transmit impulses to contract muscle fibers, and possibly reduce the frequency of soft-tissue injuries. Most importantly, a good warm-up will improve your ability to be centered: physically and mentally ready to dance.

Endnotes

1. Dance is a performing art, and the ultimate goal is the communication of the meaning of the movement to an audience. This performance quality needs to be kept in mind throughout the dancer's training. For more on the meaning of movement, see chapters 9 and 10 on choreography and performance.
2. Dance technique is discussed further in chapter 2.
3. For excellent reading on the "fit dancer," please see: *Finding Balance, Fitness and Training for a Lifetime in Dance* (Princeton, N.J.: Dance Horizons/Princeton Book Company, 1991).
4. See chapter 2 for a history of the evolution of jazz dance classes.
5. Joseph Mazo, a contributing editor of *Dance Magazine*, has said that jazz dance has "a number of techniques with a wide range of styles.
6. Dance kinesiology is the science of movement pertaining in particular to dance.
7. For a definition of ballet terms see: Gail Grant, *Technical Manual and Dictionary of Classical Ballet* (New York: Dover Publications, 1976).
8. For more on stage dancing read: Richard Kislan, *Hoofing on Broadway* (New York: Prentice-Hall, 1987).
9. From Joseph H. Mazo, "Matt Mattox: The Master's Voice," *Dance Magazine*, March 1993, 70.

10. Jean Stearns, *Jazz Dance: The Story of American Vernacular Dance* (New York: Schirmer Books, 1968).
11. If you are using any copyrighted music in a classroom or performance situation, it is important to check with ASCAP (American Society of Composers and Publishers), One Lincoln Plaza, New York, NY 10023 (212) 595-3050 or BMI (Broadcast Music, Inc.), 320 W. 57th Street, New York, NY 10019 (212) 586-2000 concerning their licensing fees and procedures.
12. Jean Williams, ed., *Applied Sports Psychology*, Psychological Characteristics of Peak Performance (Mountain View, Calif.: Mayfield Pub., 1986), 125–26.
13. Jean M. Williams, ed., Robin S. Vealey, *Applied Sports Psychology*, Imagery Training (Mountain View, Calif.: Mayfield Pub., 1986), 211–12.
14. For a brief description on some relaxation techniques see: Sally S. Fitt, *Dance Kinesiology* (New York: Schirmer Books, 1988), 296–98.
15. Many great teachers of dance included breathing in their techniques as a means for expression, emphasis, and fullness of movement.
16. It is generally believed that soreness of the muscles occurs when untrained muscles work too hard, or differently. There are several possible causes, including lactic acid (waste products of exercise fuel) buildup, which stimulates nerve endings and registers as pain, or torn muscle or connective tissue. Warming up before and stretching after class may reduce the soreness from either cause.
17. Dan Wathen, "Flexibility: Its Place in Warm-up Activities," *National Strength and Conditioning Association Journal* 5 (October-November 1987): 26–27.
18. Please see part 2 of this book.
19. Please see chapter 7. Suggested body therapies and reeducating and exercise systems include the Alexander Technique, Feldenkrais, Bartinieff Fundamentals, Massage, the Nicklaus Technique, and the Pilates Method. See also: Daniel Nagrin, *How to Dance Forever: Surviving Against the Odds* (New York: William Morrow and Co., Inc., 1988) 119–64.
20. Please see chapter 4.
21. For further discussion on what should be included in a warm-up see: Berardi, Dance Horizons/Princeton Book Company, 1991 *Finding Balance: Fitness and Training for a Lifetime in Dance*, 58–60.

CHAPTER 2

Jazz Dance Technique

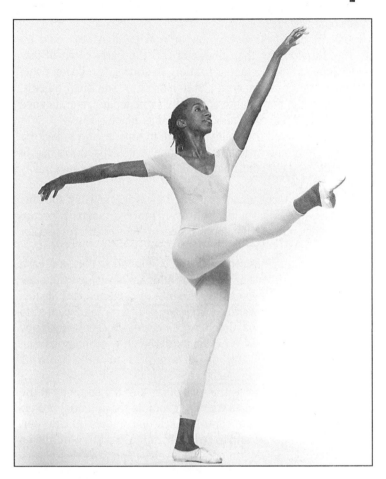

Outline

How Today's Jazz Class Developed and Why

In the late 1930s and 1940s, jazz dancing left the street corners and moved into the dance studios. "Street" dancing became a performing art and was beginning to be taken seriously as a profession.

To work in musical comedies, nightclubs, or movies, dancers could no longer celebrate the individuality that characterized the early roots of jazz dance. With professionalism came standardization. In shows, "precision dancing" was popular, and to get jobs, dancers had to learn the "routines" quickly. To learn the routines quickly, they had to speak the same language and dance the same "vocabulary." They had to develop marketable dance skills.

Skills for the chorus included the ability to move in unison, and to pick up routines fast and bring them quickly to a performance level. All dancers had to develop stamina and levels of concentration equal to the requirements of daily rehearsals and performances.

To progress beyond the chorus, dancers needed theatrical artistry, the ability to "sell" themselves, and musicality. But, even more important for the dancers, and indeed for dance itself, dancers needed *self-respect* and respect for their work.

To provide the skills and qualities required and to help "show dancers" earn respect, some outstanding teachers in the 1940s and 1950s revised the standard, classical dance class to create a new dance discipline: jazz dance. Teachers such as Jack Cole, Matt Mattox, Luigi, and Gus Giordano wanted to elevate the looked-down-upon chorus members to new levels of artistry. They worked hard to develop exercise progressions and dance combinations that would effectively train dancers' bodies while nurturing the uniquely *theatrical* style that would help their students succeed professionally.

Being selected from an audition was the goal of most of the students at the time, and jazz classes were designed as training grounds for potential professionals. Dancers needed to learn to concentrate, pick up routines quickly, perform the combinations with energy, and to *sell* their routines with more than a little exhibitionism. They also needed to take themselves and their dance very seriously to satisfy these teachers. The early classes set the style for jazz classes today. As a result, even *recreational* jazz classes have an intensity about them not found in other styles of dance classes.

These early classes were and continue to be very style dependent. For instance, one can easily tell a Cole-trained dancer from a Luigi-trained dancer. Cole's style was athletic, "into-the-floor," and heavily influenced by dances of India. In contrast, Luigi's style was pulled-up and lyrical. Their exercises reflected their dance values. Today, jazz-teaching techniques are more kinesiologically standardized, but, true to their roots, most teachers still design their classes to meet their own stylistic preferences.

Jazz is a living art form, influenced by current cultural trends and personalities. It is constantly being redefined and reinvented. As a result of this aptitude for variation, the particular bent of a given class depends upon the individual affinities of the teacher. The teacher may place emphasis on the preservation of an existing style (Siegenfeld), on gentle, correct technique (Simonson), on the relationship to the music (Luigi), on athleticism (Chandler), or on reconstructions of dances from Broadway and Hollywood (Lee Theodore of the American Dance Machine.)

Though it borrows much of its terminology from its classical counterpart, jazz dance classes do not have the universally standard exercises of ballet classes. A jazz student, for example, cannot travel from country to country switching teachers from day to day as ballet dancers sometimes do. Each jazz teacher's warm-up is different, each exercise is performed with a different emphasis, and movements are individually stylized. It sometimes takes several weeks for a new student to learn a teacher's warm-up series of exercises thoroughly enough to perform it comfortably.

This chapter reviews basic dance technique, the foundation of the modern, ballet, and jazz dance forms. It also contains a partial list of jazz moves and positions. In chapter 1 we saw that much of the terminology used in class is often from classical ballet. Particular movements, exercises, and positions may also borrow the ballet terminology, but the vocabulary is definitely stylized and recognizable as jazz. Though the teacher's style and personality remain the dominant factors in determining the exact ingredients of the class, the following movements have commonly been seen throughout the past few decades.

Basic Dance Technique

As noted in chapter 1, technique is the method one uses to accomplish the moves of dance. Today an increasing number of dancers, teachers, and choreographers understand that a knowledge of kinesiology and biomechanics can help improve the safety of the art form for the participant. Though science is not more important than art, there needs to be a well-thought-out balance of aesthetics and body mechanics to ensure proper training. The educated dancer has a basic knowledge of anatomy, physiology, and dance kinesiology.[1]

The study of dance technique is an ongoing process that the dancer never finishes nor tires of. Dancers must love to work hard and continually learn about themselves and the art form. Once good technique is achieved, the dancer strives to move even better with increasingly more ease and efficiency. Proper technique is fluid, appears effortless, and does not injure the body.

Let's begin with a review of basic dance technique.

Alignment

While in a vertical, resting position, in good alignment, the head is centered over the shoulders, the shoulders over the hips, the ribcage and pelvis are in neutral positions (neither pushed forward or back), and the abdominals engaged. The body weight is centered over the knees, which pour the weight evenly through the feet. The skeleton holds the body up, and the muscles are relaxed. Alignment should be balanced and effortless, with the abdominals working to support the torso.

Proper alignment is not merely achieved, held, then disregarded. It is also the proper placement of the body during all dance activities. It is referred to continuously as the dancer shifts through space and returned to at the end of the sequence. As the dancer moves through varying positions and actions, the knowledge of proper alignment aids in the efficiency and safety of movement. It liberates the body to move naturally and assuredly. Proper alignment is also necessary for the dancer to achieve a sense of "center."[2,3]

Alignment

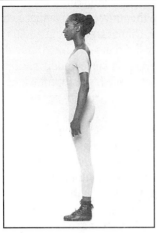
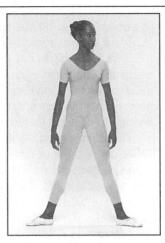

a. Alignment with the legs in parallel first position

b. Alignment with the legs in outwardly rotated (turned-out) second position.

Checklist: Alignment

- The head is centered over the shoulders, the shoulders over the hips, and the ribcage and pelvis in neutral positions.
- The abdominals are working to support the torso.
- The body weight is centered over the knees and the weight pours evenly through the feet.
- Alignment is not static, but rather a state of balance and effortlessness which is attended to continuously.
- The knowledge of proper alignment aids in the efficiency and safety of movement.
- Proper alignment is necessary to be "centered."

Turnout or Outward Rotation

Turnout is the common name given to the outward rotation of the legs at the hips. Outward rotation is a personal accomplishment. Every dancer's turnout will be slightly different in degree and appearance, determined by bone structure and the length of ligaments, tendons, and muscles in the area. The legs are outwardly rotated by engaging the muscles connecting the pelvic girdle to the femurs: the six deep rotators, the adductors, the iliopsoas, sartorius, the biceps femoris, pectineus, piriformis, and the gluteus medius.[4] Turnout should be thought of as a continuous spiraling action of the *upper thighs, not the feet*. The alignment of the pelvis will not be affected by rotation if the abdominals are engaged and are supporting the lower spine. Rather than being static, the relationship of the top of the legs to the pelvis should be constantly monitored.

Turned-out positions of
the feet

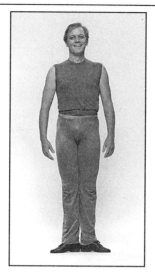

a. First position

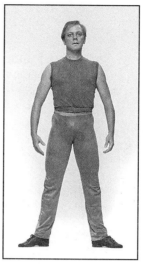

b. Second position

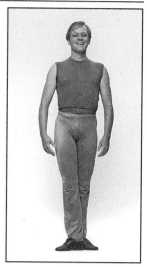

c. Third position

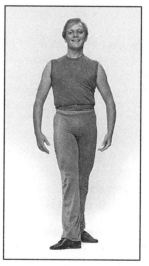

d. Fourth position

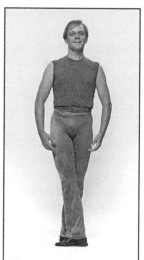

e. Fifth position

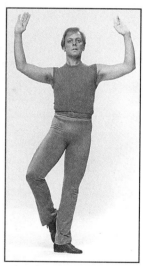

f. On one foot

Parallel and Turned-In Positions

In parallel, the legs drop from the pelvis naturally, usually about the width of the hip bones. Again the alignment of the pelvis is not affected, and the body's weight should be distributed evenly through the soles of the feet, with all the toes on the floor.

When the legs are turned-in, the femurs are rotated toward the center of the body. When executing any movement in a turned-in position, all the rules of proper alignment apply. Remember to align the knees over the toes when supporting weight.

Parallel positions

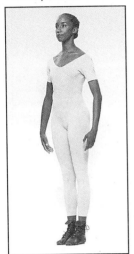

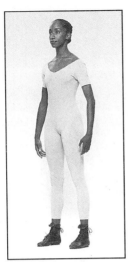

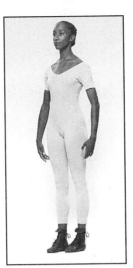

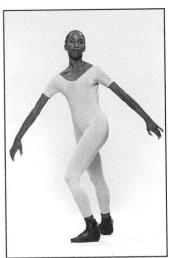

a. First position

b. Second position

c. Third position

d. An inwardly rotated thigh in demi plié.

Plié

Plié means to bend and should be thought of as a verb or action rather than a position. Plié is the softening of the knees that carries the pelvis and the body through level changes. It is basic to most dance forms. The pelvis must remain in the neutral position, and the knees aligned to bend out and over the toes. The feet should contact the floor evenly and the muscles of the ankle should be relaxed.

Demi plié (half bend) *is one of the most important dance skills because it is the preparation and ending for all jumps, most turns, and other movements.* The demi plié should be taken very seriously from the outset of dance training and executed each time properly and thoughtfully.

When executing a grand plié (full bend), it is extremely important that the dancer carries her weight well by supporting her center with the abdominals. As the pelvis girdle is lowered with a full bend of the knees, it should remain in a neutral position, neither tilting forward or backward. Grand plié helps to strengthen and stretch the legs while the dancer learns to move the pelvis through level changes with proper alignment.[5] In the second position, the heels remain on the floor and pelvic girdle is only lowered to be even with the knees. In the other positions, the heels reach toward the floor as soon as possible on the ascent.

Demi and grand plié may be done in all the outwardly rotated and parallel positions of the feet.

Relevé

Relevé means to rise or lift. In the relevé position, the heels are lifted and the weight is on the ball of the foot or feet. The ankles should be equally lengthened on both sides with all the toes on the floor. The motion of rising should not affect the turnout or alignment of the pelvis.

Plié

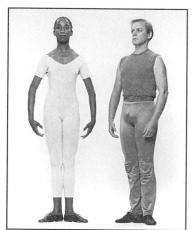

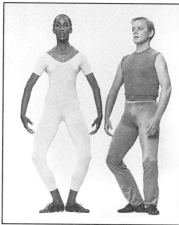

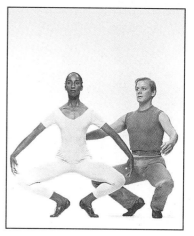

a. Turned-out first position

b. Demi-plié in turned-out first

c. Grand plié in turned out first position

Relevé

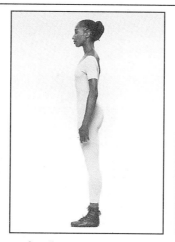

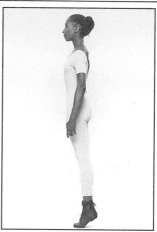

a. Standing

b. Relevé

Port de Bras

Port de bras means to carry the arms. There are several standard positions originally borrowed from ballet and now used in modern and jazz dance. Though many techniques stress that the arms are attached to the spine and should move from the torso, the alignment of the shoulders or ribcage should not be affected unless specified.

Transference of Weight

The abdominals and psoas muscle groups control the dancer's center of weight and are responsible for stabilizing the torso and pelvic area during the shift of the body weight from one foot to another. The pelvis in most cases should remain neutral, with the torso carried above it. The pelvis should move to align

Port de bras

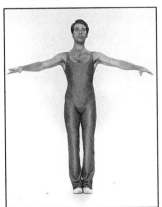 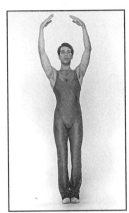 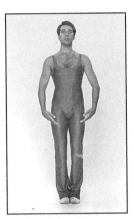 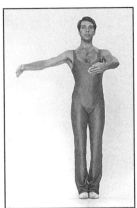

a. Arms in second position

b. Arms in high fifth position or en haut (above)

c. Arms in low fifth or bras bas (arms down)

d. Arms in the preparatory position for turning or fourth position

Transference of weight

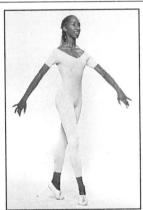 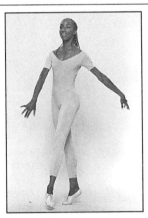 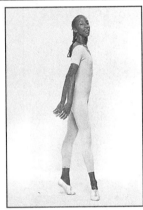

Jazz walking in relevé

a.   b.   c.

Moving forward from plié in fourth to a lunge

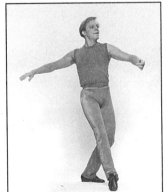 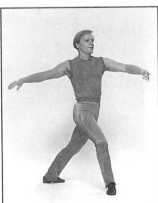

d.   e.

itself over the feet with each step. In jazz, the hips are often pushed off center. Knowing where the pelvis is and knowing how the muscles of this area work together makes controlling the transference of weight more efficient. To master this, the dancer must have an acute awareness of the muscles at the top of the legs, knowledge of alignment, and sufficient abdominal strength. Carrying the weight through space is one of the dancer's most basic and important skills.

 Checklist: Dance Technique

- Alignment should be effortless and balanced with the abdominals holding the only tension. The ribcage and pelvis are in neutral positions.
- Proper alignment aids in the efficiency and safety of movement and liberates the body to move naturally and assuredly.
- The legs turn out from the hip by using the muscles at the top of the thighs.
- Demi-plié is one of the most important dance skills since it is the beginning and end to every jump, most turns and other movements.
- Demi-plié and grand plié should be executed with the knees over the toes, the torso and pelvis in neutral positions, and the fullest turnout when appropriate.
- Body weight should be distributed evenly across the foot both when standing on flat feet and in relevé.
- Carry the arms through their positions keeping the shoulders and ribcage from raising excessively.
- To master transference of weight, the dancer must have an acute awareness of the muscles at the top of the legs, knowledge of alignment, and sufficient abdominal strength.
- Carrying the weight through space is one of the dancer's most basic and important skills.

Vocabulary

Now let's take a look at some common moves or the vocabulary of jazz dance. Many are ballet steps that have been stylized over the past decades and adopted into the jazz idiom. Because of the ever-changing vocabulary and inventiveness of jazz dance, a definitive list could never be assembled. For a more complete listing of ballet terms, however, please refer to a classical ballet dictionary.[6]

Jazz Walks

There are as many types of jazz walks as there are personalities. They are traveling steps, simple walking, with any stylized use of the shoulders, accentuated hip motion or position of the torso.

Jazz walks with the shoulders in opposition
High level on relevé

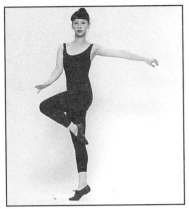

a.

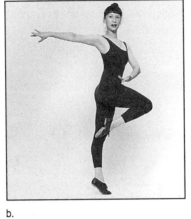

b.

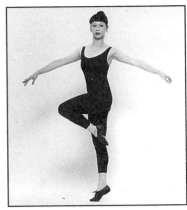

c.

Medium level

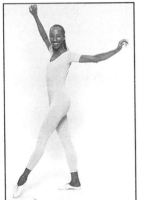

a.

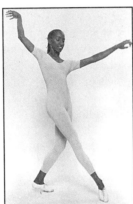

b.

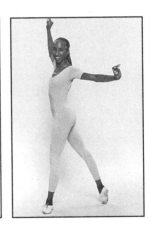

c.

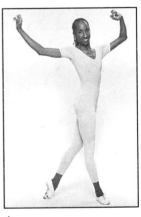

d.

Low level in plié

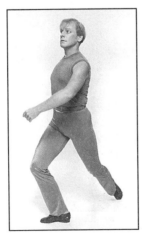

a.

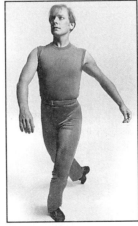

b.

Jazz Turns

Many jazz turns are stylized versions of those found in ballet, such as a pencil (soutenu) turn, an outside (en dehors) turn, or a chain (chaîné) turn. All of these examples begin and turn on the left foot, though note the direction of each turn.

Jazz turns

Pencil turn: the right leg sweeps behind the left, turning to the right

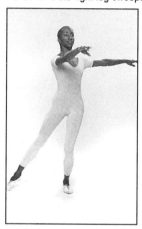 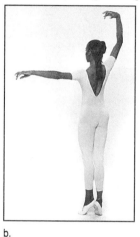 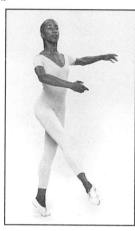 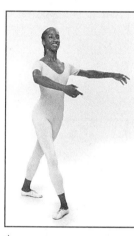

a.   b.   c.   d.

Outside turns

Outside turn: the right toe meets the left ankle also turning to the right

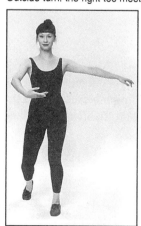 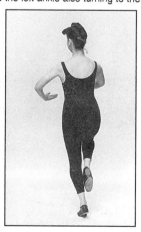 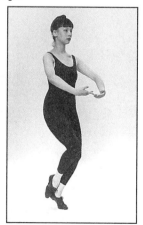 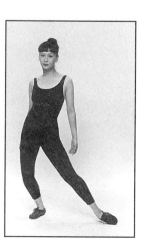

a.   b.   c.   d.

Inside turn

Inside (en dedans) turn: the right toe touches the left ankle but turns to the left

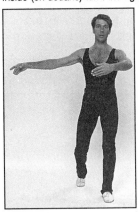

a.

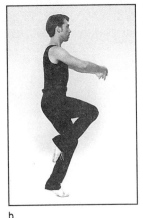

b.

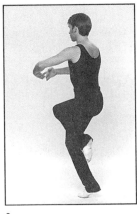

c.

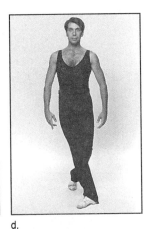

d.

Chain (chainés)

Chain turn: the feet meet in parallel first position, turning to the left)

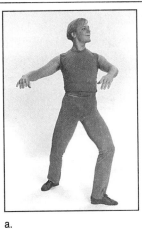

a.

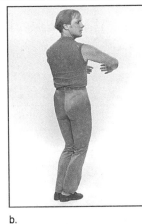

b.

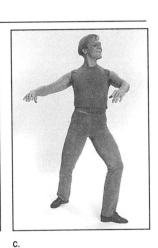

c.

Elevations

Leaps begin on one foot and land on the other foot. Hops begin and land on the same foot, and jumps begin and land on both feet. Remember correct placement of the pelvis and use of the abdominals will help in the height and landings of any elevation.

Extensions

Often called kicks or battements. Battement is the French ballet term for beat. Grand battement is a large beat, or the exercise in which the leg is raised from the hip into the air, with the knee straight. They can be done to the front, side, or back, usually without distortion to the alignment of the pelvis.

Elevations

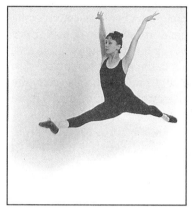 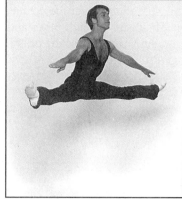 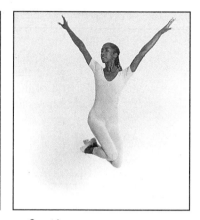

a. Forward leap   b. Side leap   c. Squat jump

Extensions

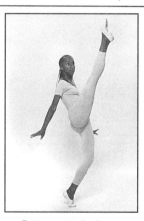 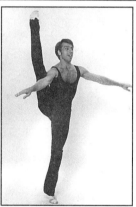 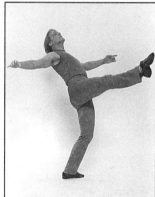

a. Battement to the front on   b. Battement to the side   c. Layout
    forced arch (the standing
    leg in plié on relevé)

Pas de bourreé

Pas de bourreé: a three-step movement with many variations (twenty-two variations are listed in Gail Grant's *Technical Manual and Dictionary of Classical Ballet*). One commonly used in jazz is to step to the side with the right foot, cross the left foot behind the right, then step side with the right foot again. Pas de bourreé may be done traveling to the side, front or back, turning, or covering a great deal or minimal amount of space. It is used as a connecting step in many combinations.

Contractions

A contraction is a very strong use of the abdominals that hollows out the front of the body. It should be considered a *lengthening of the back versus a shortening of the front.* The contraction lengthens the lumbar region of the spine, improving flexibility, and develops strength in the abdominals. Strength in this area is necessary to master control over the center of weight and control over moving the body through space. Though other abdominal work will be done in class (sit-ups, roll-ups, etc.), the contraction offers a way to build strength in this area while standing. A full contraction and release aids in the forward and backward tilt of the pelvis, a move used often in jazz dance. Contractions also help the dancer to gain control over his or her center. Mastery of the contraction will aid the dancer in establishing balance and equilibrium.

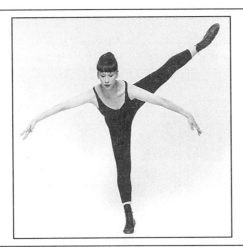

A contraction with an attitude to the side

Summary

Once jazz dancing left the street corners and moved into dance studios, "street" dancing became a performing art. To become a professional in musical comedies, nightclubs, or movies, dancers had to develop marketable dance skills. Jazz dance classes were designed as training grounds for potential professionals.

Outstanding teachers such as Jack Cole, Matt Mattox, Luigi, and Gus Giordano revised the classical dance class to create a new discipline called jazz dance.[7] The early classes set the style for jazz classes today by developing exercise progressions that would effectively train dancers' bodies while nurturing the uniquely *theatrical* style that would help students succeed professionally. Though more standardized today, jazz teaching techniques are designed by individual teachers to meet their own stylistic preferences.

Each jazz teacher's warm-up is different, and it may take several weeks to learn a teacher's warm-up thoroughly. Yet there are some common elements and vocabulary that have survived the continuous changes over time. The basics of dance technique, however, are the same in the forms of modern, ballet, and jazz.

Endnotes

1. For additional information on the science of human motion, please refer to the suggested reading in the bibliography.
2. For more on alignment please see:
   Daniel Lewis, *The Illustrated Dance Technique of Jose Limon* (New York: Harper & Row, 1984), 37.
   Watkins and Clarkson, *Dancing Longer, Dancing Stronger*, 19.
3. For more on "center," please see chapter 1.
4. An excellent guide to the muscles of the hip can be found in: Fitt, *Dance Kinesiology*, 137–68.
5. The necessity (beyond tradition) of the grand plié has been a topic of debate for many years. Grand plié must be done cautiously as hyperflexion of a weight-bearing knee puts stress on the knee joint. There are alternate methods to safely strengthen the thighs. Some are listed in chapter 5.
6. See: Anna Paskevska, *Ballet: From the First Plié to Mastery* (Princeton, N.J.: Dance Horizons/Princeton Book Company, 1990) or
   Gail Grant, *Technical Manual and Dictionary of Classical Ballet* (New York: Dover Publications, 1976).
7. Please see What is Jazz Dance, chapter 8.

The Jazz Dance Class: A Model

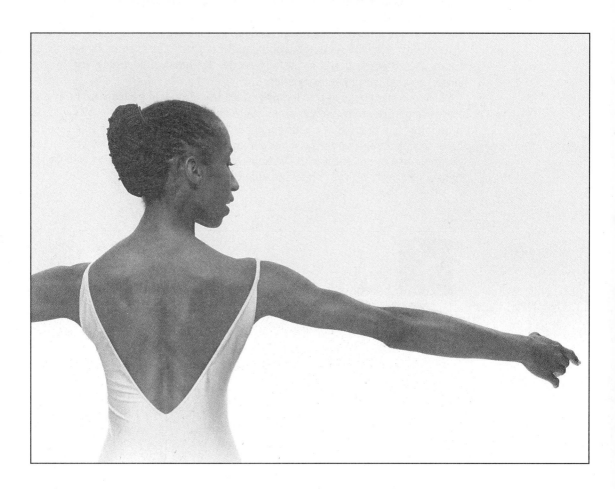

Outline

Now we are ready to proceed to the jazz dance class. Most classes, regardless of stylistic differences, are divided into elements. The order of the elements on the following list corresponds to the order in which they are often executed. The order is common but not absolute, although this sequence may optimize the learning effects of the class. Ideally one should raise the body temperature slowly, tax the muscles for strength training, then stretch for the greatest results in flexibility. Aerobic training to complete the warm-up is followed by specificity training, and when the body is fully ready, the most challenging part of the class, the long combination, is offered.

The completeness of this list presumes the class will be from an hour and forty-five minutes to two hours in length. A shorter class does not provide ample time for all the technique training, skill development, and dancing that need to be accomplished. If your classes are shorter, be sure to analyze what is being taught and supplement it with the appropriate workout. Chapters 1 and 4 may help you to evaluate your class and suggest additional exercises.

Checklist: Common Elements of the Class

- Warm-up   General (large muscles groups)
  Finer tuning (smaller muscle groups)
  Strengthening exercises
  Flexibility exercises
  Endurance conditioning
  Isolations
- Specific skill development
- Short combinations and movements for coordination and skill-building
- Longer combinations and choreography
- Cool-down
- Reverence

The jazz warm-up (the first six elements) is often lengthy and done in a continuous fashion so that the body stays warm and flexible. It usually lasts thirty to forty-five minutes, and it is here that most of the bodywork gets done. The above elements are further divided so the dancer can work on individual movements slowly and carefully. General movements for large muscle groups progress into specific and more refined activities. Centering and alignment should be the first considerations. Once these are established, the dancer will be able to better concentrate on technique, strengthening, and flexibility.

The warm-up is usually arranged to music, remains the same week to week, and is learned over a period of time. While the dancers learn to do the exercises with more proficiency, they will develop empathy for the accompaniment and work on musicality. In jazz dance, the music often helps to motivate and inspire the dancer to move. Learn to listen while moving. Dancers should also try to imitate the attitude and characteristics of their instructor, as each may have his or her own approach to movement. In this way, the warm-up serves the dual purpose of training the body and teaching the jazz dance style.

Physical Training

Ideally a jazz warm-up should include all the exercises (stretches and toners) that are necessary for training the body to dance, but in practice it cannot address every individual's needs. As discussed in chapter 1, the dancer must take ultimate responsibility for his/her own warm-up. Often in jazz, isolated body parts move to accent the music,[1] which is sometimes very percussive, so the body has to be prepared to move powerfully. The muscles must be toned and pliable. The torso must be strong enough to stabilize forcefully moving limbs and to protect the back. Standard calisthenic-type exercises, such as sit-ups, curl-downs, and push-ups, are sometimes included in a warm-up, but they are usually "choreographed" to make them more interesting and stylistically appropriate.

Style Training

During the warm-up you also have time to learn the stylistic details of posture and "line" that are important to the genre of jazz dance. A dancer's line is the ideal design of the body in space. The tilt of the head, a rolled-in shoulder, and a flexed foot are details of a particular *line*. *Style*, you remember from chapter 1, is the distinction given to the dance by a character or school. It is "the specific manner of expression peculiar to a work, a period, or a personality. It implies the purposeful and consistent choice of expressive ingredients to achieve a characteristic manner."[2]

Being able to adopt and pick up a style quickly is one of the goals of taking a jazz dance class. Try to emulate the attitude and flow of the teacher, and *dance* the warm-up sequence almost as if it were a performance. This will help you develop performance capabilities as soon as possible.[3] Maintaining a performance level of concentration throughout an entire forty-five-minute warm-up requires a great deal of focus, stamina, and practice. By *performing* the warm-up, dancers develop these attributes at the same time they are learning the basics of technique.

Being in an appropriate frame of mind is extremely important to maximize learning. Review the section on mental preparation in chapter 1, then read through the following notes. Adhering to them will increase your chances of having a successful class.

Checklist: Preparing for a Successful Class

- Begin the warm-up slowly, allowing your body time to adjust to vigorous movement.
- Concentrate on the music as well as your body as you warm-up.
- Develop your levels of concentration and stamina slowly and consistently. To avoid burnout, do not expect to be able to complete the whole warm-up immediately.
- Observe *how* you learn movement. Some dancers watch the teacher and then move, some move along with her as she demonstrates, some need to count, some need to hear the music. All methods are valid, but one might be more right for you. Experiment.
- Do not feel pressured to push yourself to a level beyond your capability. Your concentration should be on your own dancing—not on someone else's technical achievements.
- Once you know the combination, play with it. Develop an independent movement style as well as the ability to conform.[4]
- Don't be shy. This is a dance style with roots in a culture that celebrated the inhibition of the individual's creativity within a group. (See chapter 8.)
- When you're not dancing, you can and should still participate by watching (a viable learning tool) or clapping and vocally supporting the other dancers when appropriate.
- Try not to be competitive. It can be very damaging if you allow others in the class to intimidate you. Do the best you can and *enjoy it*.

Warm-up Sets

Many contemporary jazz teachers choreograph the first six elements into a series of exercise "sets."[5] Each set has four or five exercises that have something in common: either they work the same general body part (such as the large or smaller muscle groups, upper back, hamstrings), emphasize the same style of movement (percussive, lyrical), need the same kind of music (isolations), or take place in the same space (floor, barre, center floor, etc.).

Since a set usually lasts the length of the music it is done to, if it is well-choreographed, each set can seem like an individual dance, with a beginning, middle, and end. The advanced dancer has the opportunity to merge the physical and stylistic techniques of the warm-up and play with the phrasing and performance motivations inspired by the music.

In between sets in beginning classes, one typically has a few seconds to drop the performance level and relax. In some classes, the dancers often applaud between sets to reward themselves for their effort and to encourage their peers, but the class must proceed consistently enough to build stamina and concentration.

General Warm-up (Large Muscle Groups)

The first movements of a jazz class are for the larger muscle groups and facilitate the general warming and integrating of the body. These exercises should be done slowly and thoughtfully, with concentration on engaging the abdominal muscles to support the torso and keeping the pelvis in a neutral position. Pay attention to the turnout muscles of the upper thigh and to the proper placement of the feet.[6] Remember, the initial concern of any class should be the attainment of proper alignment.

Proper Alignment. A Review

The head is centered over the shoulders, the shoulders over the hips, the ribcage and pelvis are in neutral positions (equal in the front and back), and the abdominals engaged. The body weight is centered over the knees, which pour the weight evenly through the feet. The skeleton holds the body up, and the muscles are relaxed. Alignment should be balanced and effortless, with the abdominals supporting the lumbar spine.

Proper alignment is not achieved and held but is also the proper placement of the body while moving. It is referred to continuously as the dancer shifts through space and returned to at the end of the sequence. Proper alignment aids in the efficiency and safety of movement and liberates the body to move naturally and assuredly. Proper alignment is necessary for the dancer to achieve a sense of "center."

This first set of exercises should be done with the quality of a yawn. It is a general "waking up" for the entire body. It may consist of demi pliés, balances, and easy stretches. (Irene Dowd suggests reaching to the extreme positions to begin to warm the body, gently stretching the hands and feet as far as possible, in as many directions away from center.[7]) The objective is to get in touch with the body. During the first set, the dancer should shift his or her focus from anything outside class to the business at hand. Concentration is the key to a successful class.

Fine Tuning (Smaller Muscle Groups)

The next element, for smaller or finer muscle groups, continues to warm the body more specifically. The dancer should be totally focused on his/her body by now and be applying all that he or she knows about technique. Examples of finer tuning include tendus, degagés, ronds de jambe,[8] articulations of the feet and shoulders, and exercises turning the legs in and out. You will be concentrating on standing on one or the other leg with the proper alignment and lengthening the spine with energy.

The set will be done alternating right and left feet, first working in parallel positions, then outwardly rotated. Initially the arms may be in a relaxed state, naturally hanging beside the body. As proficiency with the legs increases, choreographed movements of the arms may be added to enhance coordination training. Pay attention to the alignment of the pelvis and support the spine by engaging the abdominals. Continue to breathe evenly and deeply, and image the muscles loosening and becoming more energized.

Strengthening Exercises

Once the body is warmed up, it can be pushed to perform exercises that will tire and tax the muscles. It is by pushing the normal limits that one develops increased muscle strength. Dancers must do abdominal exercises frequently to maintain the strength of the torso. Strength in this area is very important because it stabilizes the body and protects the spine when the body is thrown into unusual postures and movements. Strengthening exercises include: contractions and sit-ups for the torso, port de bras for the arms, and hinges, lunges, developpés,[9] and pliés for the legs.

As discussed previously, the reason for the plié exercises is to develop strength in the legs and to learn to carry the pelvis through level changes without anterior and posterior tilts. Simultaneously, you will work on outward rotation where applicable and strengthening of the inner thighs. Additional balances should also be included in this set.

As with all the warm-up, this set may incorporate both parallel and outwardly rotated positions. The exercises may be separated by a choreographed set of arm movements, slow turns, or walks.

Follow these exercises with a series of choreographed sit-ups and push-ups, making sure to vary and increase the exercises in order to progress. Jazz dance uses many acrobatic moves that transfer weight to parts of the body other than the feet. Be sure to do strengthening exercises for all the major muscle groups that will be used in the choreography. (For additional strength work, please see chapter 5.)

Flexibility Exercises

One key to a dancer's development is the creation of balance between strength and flexibility in as many areas of the body as possible. (Flexibility is defined as the range of motion around the joints.)[10] Once body temperature has been raised one or two degrees by the general warm-up and strengthening exercises, the body will be able to stretch more effectively.

In a class situation, it is often difficult to create the ideal environment for increasing flexibility. Flexibility exercises should be done in a relaxed, comfortable, and noncompetitive manner. The energy of the jazz class may, however, keep dancers from totally relaxing. The constraints of staying within musical phrasing may also inhibit a sufficiently thorough stretch. Remember to breathe, visualize, and concentrate without regard to the demands of the music or the teacher. Music with a slower tempo facilitates the relaxation needed for proper, thorough stretching and makes for a calmer dancer. The dancer should feel free to lengthen and shorten certain stretches—regardless of the musical phrasing—to ensure safer stretching.

All major muscle groups should be properly stretched, and the dancer must pay careful and special attention to his/her body. Supplement the class routine with whatever other exercises that are necessary. Within the framework of the class, be careful to monitor your own muscles and be sensitive to what your body needs. *Remember the key words for stretching are slowly and carefully.* Bouncing or sudden stretching may cause undue stress on body parts and result in injury. Relax and keep breathing. A good general rule for stretching is to be passive in the position on your inhale and stretch on the exhale. Stretch for at least thirty-two counts in each position to a slow tempo. The following are examples of stretches you may do in class. Ideally you should be given thirty to sixty seconds to stretch in each position.

All the stretches may be choreographed into a flexibility set and intermingled with other floor work.

Hamstring stretch

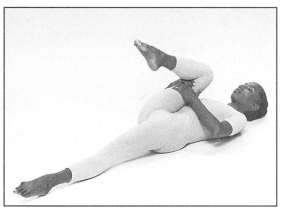 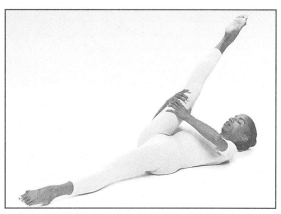

a. The spine will be in a straight line from the head to the toe of the extended foot. (Make sure to hold the thigh behind, rather than on top of, the knee.)

b. Relax the bent leg and lengthen the stretched leg. Slowly extend the flexed knee to a long position as you exhale. Repeat on the other leg.

Hip flexor stretch

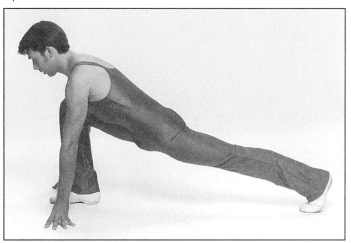

This exercise is for the muscles in front of the hip and the iliopsoas group. The flexed knee must be over, not in front of the foot, with the shin perpendicular to the floor. The body weight may be supported in part by the hands. The extended leg should be in parallel, the hip dropping gently toward the floor. Repeat on the other leg.

Quadriceps stretch

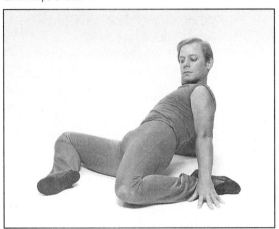

This position should only be used for stretching the quadriceps in the front of the thigh. Be sure to adjust the legs so no pressure or discomfort is felt in either knee or hip.11 The back of the hip of the leg being stretched should not be forced toward the floor. The front leg must remain bent to avoid strain on the lower back. Inhale deeply and lower the same arm as front leg to the floor behind you and put weight on it. Exhale, pull the abdominals in as far as possible and look toward the quadricep you are stretching.

Calf stretches

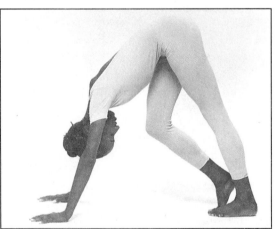

In this position, if you shift the weight forward onto the hands, you'll feel the stretch closer to the Achilles tendon. If the weight is pushed back, more on the feet, the stretch will move into the middle of the gastrocnemius. Stretch one leg at a time, then both together. The abdominals must be working the entire time to support the back.

Inner thigh stretch

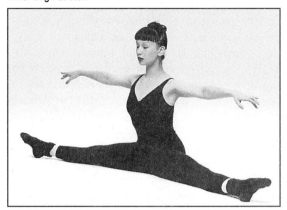

a.

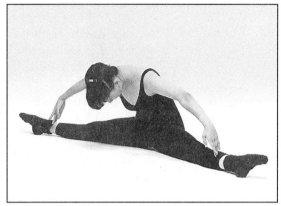

b.

Reaching forward with the head in a direct line from the spine is one way to stretch in this position, or you may choose to reach the top of the head toward the floor with a curved spine. Whichever you choose (some of each is best), remember to work the abdominals, try to keep the knees directed toward the ceiling, and lengthen the legs without locking the knees.

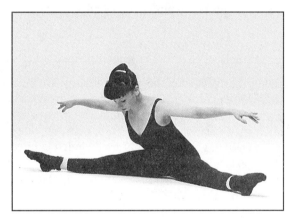

c.

Endurance Conditioning

Endurance (or aerobic) conditioning is probably the most overlooked element of the jazz dance class. (Please see chapters 1 and 4.) Simply, aerobic conditioning uses oxygen and is only accomplished when the body is pushed for a sustained period of time to raise the heart rate to 60 percent to 80 percent of its maximum.[13] Most classes rely on the repetition of the longer combinations for an aerobic workout, though due to their brevity, this is rarely sufficient for good endurance training. Sometimes rehearsals will be adequate if they are done conscientiously, making sure to run a longer piece (twelve to twenty minutes) full-out *at least* once all the way through without stopping. Most often the dancer will have to supplement his training with additional aerobic training. The benefits of this type of training are increased energy and reduced fatigue. Most dancers realize how helpful this can be to meet the daily regimen of classes and rehearsing.

The endurance set of your class may be simple exercises repeated over and over. It may include steps such as kick-ball-change, step jumps, chassés and grapevines.[14] An endurance set can be progressively increased by jumping higher on the elevations, by doing two rotations in the turning sections, by doubling the tempo of sections during repetitions, and by covering increasingly more space during the routine. Using the arms with energy and especially in positions higher than the head is very effective. A progressive workout continues to challenge the dancer and continually results in increased endurance capabilities and strength. The more you put into it, the more challenging and beneficial this set will be.

By now the heart rate should be elevated and the body temperature raised one or two degrees. It is the perfect time to stretch, as the muscles are completely warm and able to elongate fully. Then move immediately into the next series of movements. This will further the aerobic effects and increase the stress on the muscles, ultimately resulting in an improved capacity for work. Continuing to move may also reduce the incidence of injury because the muscles won't be given any time to cool and stiffen.

Isolations

Isolations, the alphabet of the jazz vocabulary, are the movements of a single area or joint. These exercises develop coordination and articulation of the body parts: head, shoulders, ribcage, hips, feet. Isolations usually carry a body part from the center-aligned position to a side, front, back, up, down, or diagonal position and return to center again. Variations are included in most jazz dance classes.

When executing each move, try to be as specific and clear as possible. While moving one body part, make sure the rest of the body is in good alignment and free of tension. Each time you return to center, check your alignment and apply this concept to the entire set. Also, you may prepare for spotting by focusing clearly in each direction while doing isolations of the head. (Spotting is a method of using the head and eyes while executing turns.)

You have completed the first six elements, or the warm-up section of the class. Review chapter 1 on an adequate warm-up. Then go through the following questions to see whether your warm-up was successful.

Checklist: Was Your Warm-up Successful?

- Is your heart rate elevated?
- Has your body temperature increased?
- Are your muscles stretched and the joints pliable?
- Do you feel "centered," physically and mentally ready to dance full-out?

Specific Skill Development

Completion of the warm-up prepares the dancer to confidently practice specific skills. During this portion of the class, individual movements that will later be put into longer combinations of choreography can be rehearsed and perfected. This work is often done in the center or "across the floor" either traveling diagonally or straight across the room. All movement should be done on both sides, beginning with one foot, then repeating the movement beginning with the other foot.[15] Use the visualization techniques in chapter 1 to correctly imagine yourself doing each movement during the teacher's demonstration or while others are taking their turns. Among other moves, during this set the dancer can expect to practice: leg extensions (a series of grand battements or kicks which may be done to the front, side, or back, both through developpé and with a straight leg. Extensions may also be done with the supporting leg in plié), elevations (leaps and hops across the floor using various positions and preparations), and turns (outside or en dehors, inside or en dedans, pencil turns, three step turns and chaînés).

During this set, dancers will probably have the opportunity to move as a group and individually. Observing classmates will reinforce your learning and train your eye. Do not let your attention or focus drop.

Short Combinations

"Specificity of training" is the theory that the best way to train for an activity is to do the activity. By this theory's logic, dancing should occupy the majority of the dancer's training. Hence the remainder of the class will be devoted to the linking of movements into sequences. Short combinations are for the development of the mind-body relationship (neuromuscular coordination)[16] and the continued development of skill and style.

While working on short combinations and phrases, try using the psychoneuromuscular theory (see chapter 1). As others are taking their turns, notice the movements being done and try to imagine yourself doing them. Imagine how it *feels* to do them correctly and which parts of the body will be engaged in the movement. When it is your turn, you will already have had a virtual rehearsal.

Short phrases may be repeated as many times as necessary to give students a sense of accomplishment and mastery. The phrases should be done on both sides to balance the training. They may link chassés, pivot turns, kicks, and leaps. Usually three to four moves are executed in a row. Some examples are listed below. All of these travel across the floor and should be repeated as many times as space allows. All take eight counts to complete.

- Step forward onto the left foot and battement the right leg to the front, arms in second position. Step on the right, step behind the right with the left and side again with the right (pas de bourreé).[17] Step onto the left, pushing the left hip forward and pivot turn 180° to the right. Step left and pivot again. Repeat.
- Step onto the right foot, left arm forward, right arm to the side. Execute an en dehors turn, in a parallel plié position, meeting hands at the sternum, the elbows bent. Step onto the left foot, relevé, and bring the right toe to

the left knee in parallel. The left arm will reach forward, the right arm will reach back, both at shoulder level. Step forward, right, left, right executing a three step turn to the right. Step left then repeat from beginning.

- Starting with the right foot, jazz walk four steps, arms swinging in opposition to the legs. Step right and face front, join the left foot to the right, both legs in parallel first position plié. Sweep the right arm side up to second position, palm flexed and to the right. Half circle the head right, down and to the left, then down and to the right.
- Chassé forward with the right foot, with the left arm forward and the right arm to the side. Step onto the left and execute an en dehors turn. Step forward onto the right foot and jump forward landing with the feet together, the arms flexed at the elbow directly to the sides of the body. Squat jump off both feet traveling left. During the second jump, bring the legs up under the backside, thighs parallel to the floor, arms straight overhead.

Long Combinations

Most dancers wait eagerly for this section of the class. It is during this time that one really gets to dance and use all the technique he or she has been practicing. The long combination should be repeated as many times as necessary to ensure a proper workout and to give the dancers enough time to master the movements of the choreography. Dancers should emulate the style of the choreography presented, and then, if given the chance to do so, embellish it with a style of their own. Careful execution of all the warm-up exercises will prepare the dancer for this set.[18]

Cool-down

Cool-down, the gradual reduction of stress on the body, has long been a neglected aspect of the dance class. Like the need for aerobic conditioning, it is slowly gaining respect. The cool-down period may be as important as the warm-up.[19] Decreasing the intensity of the exercise, stretching, and slowing down may prevent blood from collecting in the active areas and may also prevent muscle soreness later. The best time to stretch is when body temperature is elevated, so it is sensible to end class with a cool-down period that includes flexibility exercises. Since most teachers like to end on a high note, the responsibility of doing an effective cool-down may be left to the student. Attention should be paid to those muscles that were most taxed during the class. Slow, smooth stretches of the hamstrings, calves and ankles, shoulders, quadriceps, and the lower back are recommended.

Reverence

A wonderful tradition in most dance classes is the final element of reverence. It is proper etiquette for the teacher to thank the students and musicians, and for the students to thank the teacher by way of pausing momentarily and clapping. Many forms of dance also include a formal bow to the teachers and musicians, like the curtsy of dancers in a ballet class. This recognition is a demonstration of the mutual appreciation of both the givers and takers of the dance class.

Summary

Jazz dance classes, regardless of stylistic differences, are usually divided into elements in an order to best prepare the body for movement. The class progresses from warming the larger muscle groups to warming smaller, finer groups. Strengthening and flexibility exercises precede the aerobic conditioning and isolations that complete the warm-up. Centering and alignment should be the focus of the warm-up. Once these are established, the dancer will be able to better concentrate on technique, strengthening, and flexibility. The warm-up serves the dual purpose of training the body and teaching the jazz dance style. The first six elements are followed by specificity training and short combinations, and when the body is fully ready, the most challenging part of the class, the choreography, is offered.

Being in an appropriate frame of mind is extremely important to maximize learning. Begin slowly, allowing your body time to adjust to vigorous movement. Concentrate on the music as well as your body as you warm-up. Your concentration should be on your personal development. Work with integrity and a positive attitude, and most of all, enjoy yourself.

Endnotes

1. Isolated body parts used as visual rhythm can be seen particularly in the choreography of Bob Fosse and Jack Cole and in the styles of pop performers Paula Abdul and Michael Jackson.
2. The definition of style from Richard Kislan, *Hoofing on Broadway* (New York: Prentice-Hall, 1987), 183.
3. In a jazz dance class, the ultimate goal is performance. Rehearsing performance qualities and attitudes should be incorporated into the training as soon as possible.
4. The plot of the long-running Broadway show *A Chorus Line* concerns a dancer that made it out of the chorus line and into solo roles. At this particular Broadway audition, all she wants is a job, any job, but the choreographer wonders whether she can still *conform* to the chorus.
5. In Luigi's technique, the full (forty-five minute) warm-up begins with a brief (five minute) "warming-up" period called the pre-warm-up. The emphasis would be on relaxation and breathing. The imagery would be of a ragdoll and any thoughts of "proper" dance line avoided, no straight knees and no pointed feet allowed, no tension at all.
6. Review chapter 2 on dance technique.
7. From a workshop on *Warming-up* by Irene Dowd at the *Science and Somatics of Dance* Seminar. Temple University, February 1991.
8. *Tendu* means stretched. The working foot slides from the beginning position along the floor to a full point. Both knees must be kept straight. When it reaches the point, it then slides back to the starting position. There is no transfer of weight. The position of the pelvis must not be affected. Tendu may be done in parallel, in outwardly rotated positions, and in demi plié. *Degagé* is a tendu that is disengaged or leaves the floor. As the foot comes to a full point, the toe is lifted slightly from the floor. *Rond de jambe* means circle the leg. The leg is stretched (tendu) either to

the front or back and traces a half circle along the floor to the opposite position before closing in either first or third position.

9. *Developpé* means to develop and is a movement in which the gesturing leg is drawn up so that the toe is at the other knee, and slowly extended to an open long, position in the air. Developpés are done to acquire balance and strength. The hips are always kept level and square to the direction the dancer is facing.

10. See chapter 6 for more on flexibility.

11. This stretch is examined more closely in J. Alter, *Surviving Exercise* (Boston: Houghton Mifflin Company, 1983), 69–70.

12. See J. Alter, *Stretch and Strengthen* (Houghton Mifflin Company, 1986) for ideas on stretching safely without causing discomfort to the lower back.

13. In addition to cardiovascular fitness, aerobic exercise provides one of the best methods of weight control, often so crucial to the dancer. Please see cardiorespiratory conditioning in chapter 4 for more on endurance training.

14. *Kick-ball-change* is a very common connecting step in jazz in which after completing a small kick of the lower leg, the weight is shifted briefly from one foot to the other in syncopated time. There is an illustrated example on page 4 of chapter 1.

    Step jumps are simply stepping on then jumping off one foot and landing on two feet.

    Grapevine is a continuous set of steps traveling to the side where the feet alternate stepping in front then in back of each other. For example, step to the right with the right foot. Step to the right with the left crossing in front of the right. Step to the right again, and left again, this time stepping behind the right foot.

    Chassé means chased and is the action of sliding the front foot forward then pushing off into the air. The back foot simultaneously pushes off and meets the front, usually in third position (chasing the front foot). The weight is transferred quickly to the back and onto the front foot again.

15. Dance is rigorous in its attempt to train each side equally.

16. The brain sends signals of "contract" to the muscles via electrochemical pathways. Research has shown that these pathways can be developed through use. Once efficient communication pathways have been established, those pathways can be used more easily. (This explains the ease with which most of us walk.) The human brain not only recognizes previously used pathways, but it also uses old pathways for new material.

17. There are at least sixteen variations of pas de bourreé. It behooves the jazz dancer to be fluent with as many of them as possible.

18. See chapter 1, "Preparing for the Jazz Dance Class."

19. See Sally S. Fitt, *Dance Kinesiology* (New York: Schirmer Books, 1988), 319–20.

CHAPTER 4

Basic Nutrition and Cardiorespiratory Conditioning

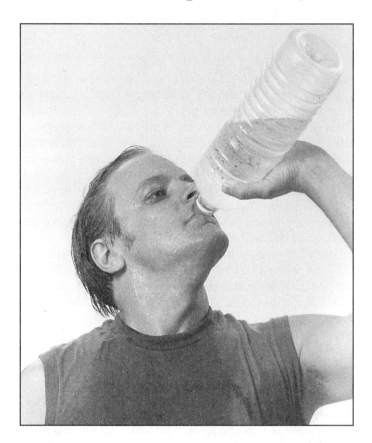

Outline

Learning to dance well mandates that you find good teachers and that you work hard. To increase your chances of having a successful career in dance or just getting what you want out of the experience of dancing, it is also useful to have some additional knowledge in related areas. Give yourself the best chance: educate yourself in the areas of nutrition and cardiorespiratory, strength, and flexibility conditioning. This chapter deals with issues in nutrition and cardiorespiratory conditioning.

Nutrition for the Dancer

Basic nutrition is necessary to our survival. While we must eat what we need to live, we may also eat what we eat for entirely different reasons. The taste, our weight and body composition, what food means to us socially and emotionally, and many other factors all contribute to what we in the twentieth century have found to be both the delights and the agonies of eating. Sensible eating requires that we know how to buy food economically and prepare it so that the nutrients are not lost. It also requires that we not get caught up in the food fads that are continually cropping up. Balancing foods to make sure we get the most from what we are eating is the key.

Dancers have special nutritional needs because they want to reduce body fat, yet still have enough strength and energy for the demands of the profession. The aesthetics of the art form requires that the performer be able to project a certain line on stage, and have enough endurance for daily classes, rehearsals, and performances. They may have to be light enough to be lifted, yet strong enough to lift others. In order to satisfy all these demands and not suffer from fatigue and weakness, the dancer must eat a balanced diet with the proper amounts of certain kinds of foods.

Eating sensibly requires that you understand the basics of nutrition. The proper nutrients (including water) must appear in the diet, and the caloric[1] intake must be sufficient to maintain a healthy weight and provide enough energy to dance. One's caloric needs change according to the activities he or she undertakes. An informed person knows the nutrients necessary for optimal functioning and puts that knowledge into practice by *setting up* and *sticking to* a proper diet. The benefits of a good diet are only realized if the nutritional habits are practiced consistently. Eating well the day of a performance or the night before class will have minimal if any effect. Above all, we must be aware of what is necessary in the way of protein, fats, carbohydrates, fibers, water, vitamins, and minerals.

Overview of the Basics

Protein is the name given to the component of food that is composed of amino acids, the building blocks of the body's tissue. About 22 such amino acids are important in human nutrition; 9 are essential and must be consumed every day. But not all amino acids occur in all protein-containing foods. We judge the quality, or "biological value" of the proteins we consume by the amount of essential amino acids in them. Though some sources of protein may have a higher "biological value" as rated by the Food and Agricultural Organization of the World Health Organization, they may not be as desirable because of the fat content of the foods they are found in. Animal sources are richest in proteins (eggs, milk, cheese, fish, poultry, beef, and pork) but are higher in fat content. Vegetable sources of proteins (legumes, wheat, corn, and nuts) have less fat but are lower in protein content. Protein supplements are often uneconomical and harmful as they may not have all the required amino acids in good quality or sufficient quantity. If we do not get enough protein, the body begins to break down tissue, usually beginning with muscle tissue, in order to release the amino acids it needs to survive.

Though dancers often believe that they need a great deal more protein in their diets, their need is actually for more carbohydrates. After we consume proteins, our digestive tract breaks them down into their component amino acids. Any amino acids in excess of what a person needs are first converted into glucose by a process called gluconeogenesis.[2] Glucose, a carbohydrate, is then used for energy. As a source for energy, this process is physiologically inefficient.

A gram of protein yields 4 calories. A healthy diet is usually made up of 10 percent to twenty percent protein.

Fats are another essential nutrient. They insulate nerves and tissue and function in transporting some of the vitamins through the body. Fats break down into fatty acids. The three major kinds of fat are: *saturated, monosaturated,* and *polyunsaturated.*

Saturated fats are generally hard at room temperature, such as animal fats, egg yolks, butter, and whole milk products. These fats bear primary responsibility for raising blood cholesterol levels and hardening the arteries and should be minimized. Current recommendations call for no more than 10 percent saturated fats in the diet, and some believe this may be too much.

Monosaturated fats, such as olive oil and peanut oil, have not generally been thought to promote hardening of the arteries and may in fact protect against arterial hardening by increasing the level of high density cholesterol in the blood. Current recommendations call for 10 percent of our diets to be monosaturated fats.

Polyunsaturated may not be as harmful as saturated fats. Generally liquid at room temperature, they are found most often in vegetable sources such as corn oil, safflower oil, and linseed oil. It is suggested that 10 percent of our diets be polyunsaturated fats.

Fats must have oxygen available to be used as fuel, providing energy in long-term, low intensity endurance situations. The absolute maximum consumption of fat should not exceed 30 percent of our total caloric intake, and probably should be closer to 15 percent to 25 percent. A gram of fat yields 9 calories.

Carbohydrates supply the major source of energy for bodily functions and muscular exertion. They supply the energy needed during dance training, rehearsing, and performing.[3] They can be such complex molecules that our digestive tract cannot break them down, or they can be very simple, quickly digestive molecules. Both complex carbohydrates: wheat, corn, beans, and legumes, and simple carbohydrates: fruits, honey, table sugar, etc., break down into glucose for energy metabolism. In addition, some forms of complex carbohydrates, such as the cellulose found in the hulls of wheat, are fibers that aid in the excretion of waste.

Though fats and proteins can both be broken down and used for energy, carbohydrates are economical energy sources. Per gram, carbohydrates have fewer calories than fats, and they are good sources for many vitamins, making them "biologically valuable." They are the main fuel source for the central nervous system, brain, and red blood cells and are needed for complete fat breakdown. The body converts carbohydrates into energy much more quickly than fat.

Dancers and other athletes who need extra energy should increase their carbohydrate intake rather than fats or proteins. Carbohydrates may be the only energy source for the working muscles during short, heavy bouts of exercise,[4] and a high carbohydrate regimen has shown to enhance endurance performance. Athletes may be able to work three times longer on a high carbohydrate diet than on a high fat diet and twice as long as when on a mixed diet.[5]

A gram of carbohydrate yields 4 calories. Carbohydrates should constitute 55 percent to 65 percent of the total dietary intake.

Fiber, or roughage, is that part of the food we eat that is not digestible. Dietary fiber is categorized as water soluble (pectins from fruit and vegetables, oat and rice brans, and gums from the seeds of tropical plants) and water insoluble (whole wheat products, wheat bran, and fruit and vegetable skins). While most Americans consume about 4 grams of dietary fiber per day, estimates on ideal intake suggest a minimum of 20 grams per day.

There is evidence that proper fiber intake can reduce many of the major intestinal problems, from the "irritable bowel syndrome" to diverticulitis and intestinal cancers. There is also some evidence that oat bran, dried beans, pectin, and certain gums can reduce blood cholesterol.

Water is a very critical human need. Water cools the body through perspiration, it carries off waste products, and it makes up a major portion of human fluids and tissues. Fifty percent to 60 percent of the body is composed of water. Though we do get some water through food sources, especially watery vegetables and fruits, and in other fluids such as juices, the National Research Council recommends drinking approximately 8 glasses of water a day. Dancers should increase this amount depending on the amount lost through perspiration and exercise. When exercising, water should be replaced regularly as dehydration may set in long before one feels thirsty. The impact of dehydration on the cardiovascular system is quite predictable. Plasma volume is lost, and the ability to provide adequate blood flow to the skin and muscles is reduced.[6] Dehydration can cause fatigue, loss of muscular strength, irritability, and loss of coordination. Dancers with even moderate dehydration may not be able to attain maximal muscle response or maximal training effort. Most professional dancers carry water bottles with them and replenish their bodies often during class.

Remember that when water has been lost through perspiration, it is the beverage of choice to replace it with. Other fluids may contain unwanted levels of fats (such as milk), sugars (juices, sodas), caffeine (coffee, tea, sodas), or sodium. In fact, the diuretics found in coffee actually help to eliminate water from the body. Water or sodium-free seltzer is best.

Vitamins are organic compounds that are essential in small amounts for our growth and development. They often act as catalysts that cause or enable many of the body processes to occur. No evidence exists to suggest that strenuous exercise increases the body's need for vitamins, nor will amounts of vitamins in excess of the Recommended Dietary Allowance (RDA) "supercharge" the cells. Vitamins do not supply energy. But dancers on a restricted diet may want to incorporate a multivitamin into their daily nutritional intake to ensure they do get all of the essentials.[7] Lack of some vitamins may cause symptoms of mental illness, such as hallucinations associated with pellagra, a niacin-deficiency disease.[8]

Minerals are usually structural components of the body, but they, too, initiate certain body processes. The body uses many minerals, among them: phosphorus and calcium for the teeth and bones, zinc for growth, chromium for carbohydrate metabolism, and copper and iron for the blood. The RDA for minerals should be closely observed as minerals are toxic at doses many times less than those of vitamins. It is wise to try to get essential minerals from food sources in the diet.[9]

What, How Much, and When

Dancers can maintain their weight and can get their basic nutrients daily if they consume the proper amounts of a variety of foods. The balance of fats (oils, nuts, cheeses, whole milks, yogurts, and animal fats), proteins (low fat milk, meat, fish, poultry, and legumes), carbohydrates (fruit, vegetables, breads, and cereals), and the individual's metabolism[10] are the most important considerations.

Most people need 13 to 17 **calories** (kcal)[11] per pound of body weight per day in order to function normally, plus those additional kcal needed for various athletic activities.[12] A typical dance class, due to its anaerobic[13] nature will normally only use 200 to 300 kcal per hour. Though dancers are seemingly very active, unless they are doing aerobic conditioning in addition to their regular classes, they may not need more than a few hundred extra kcal a day. Therefore, a 120-pound dancer would need approximately 1,560 to 2,040 kcal a day plus 200 to 300 kcal for every additional hour of dancing. If she danced for 2 hours per day, her caloric intake should be 1,960 to 2,640 kcal.

The kcal should be divided the following way:

- 55–65 percent carbohydrates: fruit, vegetables, breads, and cereals;
- 15–25 percent fats: oils, nuts, cheeses, whole milks, yogurts, and animal fats;
- 10–20% protein: low fat milks, meat, fish, poultry, and legumes.

To determine the percentage of kcal you are consuming of fat, protein, and carbohydrates, multiply the number of fat grams eaten by 9 and the number of protein and carbohydrates by 4. Divide them by the total kcal consumed to get the percentage. Consider a diet of 67 grams of fat (x 9 kcal = 603 kcal), 325 grams of carbohydrates (x 4 = 1300 kcal), and 75 grams of protein (x 4 = 300 kcal), a total of 2,203 kcal. The balance of the percentages of the nutrients would be about right: 603 ÷ 2203 = 27%, 1300 ÷ 2203 = 59%, 300 ÷ 2203 = 14%. This is a relatively low-fat, high-carbohydrate diet. To design a diet that is rich in vitamins and minerals with the proportions above, use the chart in appendix A and remember that sensible dietary habits practiced on a continuing basis, versus only immediately before class, are the cornerstones of optimal nutrition.

When, and when to eat what, are two of the major concerns of dancers. It is a combination of psychological and physiological factors that provides the answers.

Taking a dance class is not like other "classes" in the sense that one cannot eat a substantial meal immediately before working out. Many dancers feel it is not comfortable to exert and use the muscles of the abdomen for 30 to 90 minutes after consuming a normal meal.[14] Dancers with a 1 P.M. class may not have had available time at 11:30 A.M. to eat, as it may take 1 to 2 hours for a light meal and up to 4 hours for a heavy meal to digest. Scheduling meals often becomes a problem, and many dancers resort to quick, low-nutrient, high-calorie foods or to eating most of their calories at one time during the day and nearly fasting for other parts. These erratic eating patterns lead to hunger pains (the hypothalamus telling the brain to make the stomach muscles contract as the blood sugar levels decrease) and the lowering of resistance to eat nutritionally unbalanced foods. Dips in blood sugar levels and energy also may result in the body being unable to perform at its peak.

A significant proportion of one's caloric intake should be consumed before the activities of the day to ensure that tissue needs are met during training. The consumption of the majority of calories after the cessation of exercise tends to promote lipid synthesis and may lead to the accumulation of unwanted fat.[15] Eating a high carbohydrate diet daily will be the best way to provide the continuous energy needed for dance. Easily digestible carbohydrates, like those found in whole grain bread, yogurts, and pasta, eaten in small amounts 1 to 2 hours before class may be the best way to keep from getting hungry and to avoid an upset stomach. Save high-fat proteins, harder-to-digest foods, gas-producing dried fruits, raw vegetables and beans, and water-retaining salty foods for other parts of the daily schedule.

There is also the factor of mind over matter, however, and if a dancer feels that a particular food consumed at a particular time before class or a performance is a magic ingredient for success, then eating that food is appropriate. To pacify your mind with the knowledge that your body is well fueled is one of the functions of pre-event nourishment.[16]

Remember, it is the balance of fats, proteins, carbohydrates, and the individual's metabolism that is the most important consideration for proper nutrition and weight maintenance. A "fast" metabolism basically refers to one in which the person produces a lot of excess heat and thus burns up extra calories. A "slow" metabolism may indicate less wasting of calories and a proficiency at storing excess calories as fat. The excess heat needed to burn calories is mostly generated by aerobic, or endurance-type, activities. Most dancers will have to augment their dance training with some form of endurance activity to help "burn" calories by generating heat and to maintain cardiovascular fitness. Generally, dancers on a restricted diet or trying to lose weight need a reduced-calorie, low-fat diet that is high in nutrients combined with long-duration aerobic exercise.

Losing weight can only be done by reducing the number of calories you take in or by increasing the number of calories you use. We can change the types of food we eat, the amount we consume, our eating patterns, or our exercise patterns. A combination of all four works best.

Becoming aware of your eating patterns by first charting or recording when, where, why, how much, and what you eat may enable you to consciously shift and control your eating tendencies and reduce your caloric intake. There are many ways to change the way you eat that can aid in weight loss. Reduce the number of calories from fat and alcohol and the less "biologically valuable" starches and sugars. Eat broiled fish, low-fat yogurt desserts, and salads with low-calorie dressings. Avoid fried foods and whole milk products. Drink a lot of water; not only will it help to make you feel full, but water also helps to prevent water weight gain from dehydration. Eat more slowly, use smaller portions on a smaller plate, or try five small meals instead of three normal ones. (This keeps the blood sugar at a more constant level so that the hypothalamus that controls the feeling of hunger cannot tell so readily that the stomach is becoming empty.) You can also substitute low-calorie foods for others such as carrots for cookies or poultry for meat.

The recent evidence is that effective aerobic exercise is the most important part of a weight-loss program. Sedentary dieters tend to lose more muscle than fat when they diet. Those who exercise tend to lose more fat than muscle and may raise their metabolism so that more calories are used per hour both during and after the exercise bouts. For example, running for 30 minutes or walking for 2 hours will double the number of calories you will use up during the next 6 hours. In addition, aerobic exercise will improve your cardiorespiratory condition, another aspect of fitness.

Cardiorespiratory Conditioning

As mentioned, dancers trying to lose weight need a reduced-calorie, low-fat diet combined with *long-duration, aerobic* (endurance) exercise. Endurance exercise is also needed to develop the stamina to meet the requirements of daily rehearsals and performances. Though usually not a part of formal dance training, aerobic exercise is the only way to increase cardiorespiratory fitness, or the endurance capacity of the heart and lungs. When the cardiorespiratory systems adapt to allow better use of oxygen, greater levels of activity can be sustained for longer durations of time.

Without becoming too technical, aerobic activity is the *continuous maintenance of the target heart rate* and *uses oxygen* in its generation of energy. To increase cardiorespiratory fitness and "burn" calories, the activity must be sustained for at least 12 to 30 minutes at the target heart rate (THR). Your THR is 60 percent to 80 percent of your maximum heart rate. This can be calculated by subtracting your age from 220.[17] (For example 220 − 20 = 200; 200 x 70% = 140. One hundred forty beats per minute is the THR for a 20 year old.) Low-intensity (closer to 60 percent of the THR), longer-duration exercises will burn calories the most efficiently. Maintaining slightly higher target heart rates (closer to 80 percent) will further increase one's cardiorespiratory condition. For conditioning purposes, aerobic activities should be done 3 to 4 times a week.

Excellent aerobic activities for the dancer are fast walking and low-impact aerobic dance classes. The former places a minimal amount of stress on the body, while the latter may offer the fun of a social situation plus additional strength and flexibility exercises. When beginning an aerobic dance class, however, be sure to check the qualifications of the instructor and monitor the class for a proper warm-up, good alignment counseling, and a cool-down period. (See chapters 1, 2, and 3 to review warm-up, alignment, and cool-down.)[18]

Other aerobic activities include jogging, swimming, cross-country skiing, bicycling, and hiking. Try to pick an activity that is safe and sensible and that you enjoy. A variety of activities may be the most desirable, as enjoying your training will increase the probability that you stick to it.

Whichever activity you choose, remember that 12 to 30 minutes of continuous movement at 60 percent to 80 percent[19] of your maximum heart rate 3 to 4 times a week will increase your aerobic capacity and cardiorespiratory fitness.

Finally, the body adapts very specifically to what is asked of it. Short, high-intensity bouts of exercise will produce a heart capable of that type of work. Sets of longer duration will condition the system for endurance. Endurance *specific* for jazz dancing must be developed in a jazz dance class. Aerobic activities, however, will aid in weight maintenance and overall cardiorespiratory conditioning.

 Checklist: Nutrition and Weight Control

- Basic nutrition is necessary to our survival. In order to not suffer from fatigue and weakness, the dancer must eat a balanced diet.
- Water is a critical human need. As a general rule, drink approximately 8 glasses of water a day. Dancers should increase this amount depending on the amount of water loss through perspiration and exercise.
- Vitamins do not supply energy. But dancers on a restricted diet should incorporate a multivitamin into their daily nutritional intake to ensure they are getting all the essential vitamins.
- It is wise to try to get essential minerals from food sources in the diet.
- Most people need 15 to 17 kcal per pound of body weight per day in order to function normally, plus those kcal needed for additional athletic activities.
- The kcals consumed should be divided into the following percentages: 55–65 percent carbohydrates, 15–25 percent fats, 10–20 percent protein.
- Dancers on a restricted diet or trying to lose weight need a reduced-calorie, low-fat diet that is high in nutrients combined with long-duration aerobic exercise.
- Aerobic activity is *exercise that uses oxygen during sustained activity*.
- Excellent aerobic activities for the dancer are fast walking and low-impact aerobic dance classes.

Summary

While finding good teachers and working hard are prerequisites for success in dance, overall health will support the process. Every dancer should be knowledgeable in all the areas of dance fitness, including endurance (cardiorespiratory conditioning), strength, flexibility, and coordination, in addition to having current information on nutrition.

Sensible eating patterns should be practiced on a daily basis. Balancing foods to ensure getting the most from what we eat is a key to a healthy diet.[20] The proper nutrients (including water) must be included and the caloric intake sufficient enough to maintain a healthy weight while providing enough energy for the activities undertaken. An informed person knows the nutrients necessary for optimal functioning and what is necessary in the way of protein, fats, carbohydrates, fibers, water, vitamins, and minerals. Generally, dancers on a restricted diet or trying to lose weight need a reduced-calorie, low-fat diet that is high in nutrients combined with long-duration aerobic exercise.

Endnotes

1. The calorie that we use in measuring food energy is really a kilocalorie (kcal). It is a unit of heat derived by the body from food and is equivalent to 1000 times the calorie used for measuring heat in a chemistry class. It is the amount of heat needed to raise the temperature of one kilogram of water 1 degree Celsius.
2. G. Lynis Dohm, "Protein Nutrition for the Athlete," *Clinics in Sports Medicine*, vol. 3, no. 3 (July 1984).
3. Jane M. Bonbright, "Physiological and Nutritional Concerns in Dance," *JOPERD*, November/December 1990.
4. Philip D. Gollnick and Hideki Matoba, "Role of Carbohydrate in Exercise," *Clinics in Sports Medicine*, vol. 3, no. 3 (July 1984).
5. Robert Hickson, Ph.D., "Carbohydrate Metabolism in Exercise," *The Ross Symposium on Nutrient Utilization during Exercise* (Columbus, Ohio, 1983:3).
6. David L. Costill, Ph.D., "Water and Electrolyte Requirements during Exercise," *Clinics in Sports Medicine*, vol. 3, no. 3 (July 1984).
7. Vitamins have to be absorbed to be used by the body. When selecting a vitamin supplement, choose one that contains all the necessary complements to ensure that the vitamins are absorbed.
8. Please see appendix B for a list of essential vitamins.
9. Please see appendix B for a list of essential minerals.
10. See R. Chmelar and S. Fitt, *Diet: A Complete Guide to Nutrition and Weight Control* (Princeton, N.J.: Princeton Book Co., Pub., 1990), 21.
11. A moderately active average adult has an RDA of 1,600–3,000 kcal per day depending on their sex and weight.
12. See the calorie/activity chart in appendix C.
13. The opposite of aerobic, anaerobic exercise bypasses the direct use of oxygen when breaking down molecules for fuel. This process does not metabolize fat for energy. Anaerobic exercises are shorter in duration and may range in intensity. They do not promote cardiovascular endurance.
14. Muscles of the abdomen are used continually in dance. Refer to chapters 1 and 5.
15. C. Young, L. Hutler, S. Scanlon et al., "Metabolic Effects of Meal Frequency on Normal Young Men," *Journal of the American Diet Association* 61 (1972): 391.
16. Nancy Clark, M.S., R.D., *Sports Nutrition Guidebook: Eating to Fuel Your Active Lifestyle* (Champaign, Ill.: Leisure Press, 1990).

17. Other methods of determining the Target Heart Rate may be found in C. Casten and P. Jordan, *Aerobics Today* (St. Paul: West Publishing Co., 1990).

18. For more on selecting an aerobic dance class see Casten and Jordan, *Aerobics Today*, 98.

19. You may want to begin at exercises that sustain the THR at lower percentages (60) and gradually work up to 70 percent. Well-conditioned athletes may work closer to 85 percent THR.

20. The *USDA Food Guide Pyramid* is a booklet which explains and illustrates current recommendations of servings for food groups. To order it, make a $1 check payable to the Superintendent of Documents and send it to the Consumer Information Center, Department 159-Y, Pueblo, CO 81009. Ask for Home and Garden Bulletin 249.

CHAPTER 5

Supplemental Strength Training for the Dancer

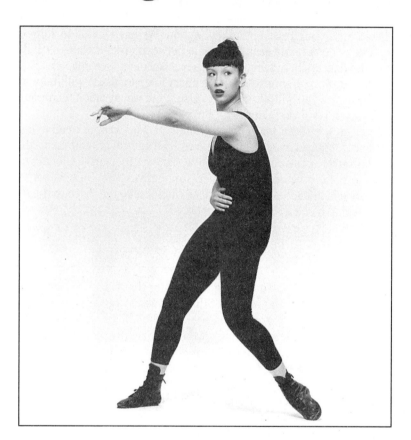

Outline

Because of time limitations, it is difficult to meet all the dance fitness goals within the class framework. To ensure that the dancer is developing in each of the fitness areas equally, often training will need to be supplemented with strength, flexibility, or aerobic activities. *Balanced* strength and flexibility in as many areas of the the body as possible is the goal of supplemental training. Often when strength and flexibility increase, so do one's technical abilities.

Variety in any training program is necessary to achieve progress; the following exercises are just a *few* suggestions. Additional exercises may be found in the books listed in the Suggested Reading Section. We have included some of those that can be done at home or in the studio between or after classes. (If not taking a class, the dancer should first do a personal warm-up [see chapter 1] and finish with a cool-down.)[1] Using the muscle chart in appendix A will help you identify which muscles you will be targeting. Using the visualization techniques described in chapter 1 will complement the work.

These exercises are meant for *noninjured* dancers who want or need to augment their training. Injured dancers, or those with structural or alignment difficulties, should first seek the counsel of a physician or other professional who can give them *personal attention and advice*. Remember that the best way to learn how to dance is to dance; these exercises cannot take the place of the formal, careful instruction of a good jazz dance class.

Supplemental Strength Training

The following exercises are just a few suggestions for the dancer who wants to increase *muscular strength*, (the ability of the muscles to generate maximum force against resistance), or *muscular endurance*, (the ability of the muscle to contract over a continued period of time). Muscles have to be worked longer (increased duration), harder (greater intensity), or more often to become stronger. Many strength exercises will be done during the jazz dance class, such as pliés and hinges for the legs, contractions for the torso and port de bras for the arms. When looking to develop more height in a leap or more leg or arm strength for a lift, strength training may be appropriate. Increased strength often is accompanied by better muscular control and coordination.

The following are some points to consider when designing a strength conditioning program.

There is a **special relationship** between strength and flexibility that the dancer should be aware of. Muscles only contract, they can't push, but there are muscles that extend to allow others to contract and vice versa. For example, when executing a flexion of the ankle, as the muscles in the front of the ankle contract, the muscles in back will release or extend. This relationship dictates that opposing muscle groups be balanced in strength and flexibility to allow the fullest and safest movement.

Overloading is the concept that the stress must continually be increased for the capacity of the body to increase. To increase *muscular strength*, the resistance must increase. To increase *muscular endurance*, the repetitions or duration must increase. The range of motion must be enhanced for flexibility to continue to develop. Add repetitions as the body adapts to the new stress.

Repetitions ("Reps") are the number of exercises done in each set. Muscular endurance will require more repetitions at lower intensities. Strength building will demand fewer repetitions at higher intensities. Be sure to work to the point of fatigue, but do not think that exhaustion will increase the benefit. Muscles need to tire to gain strength, but pushing past the point of being able to complete the exercise correctly could cause discomfort or injury. The number of repetitions depends on the muscle group being worked, larger muscle groups generally need fewer repetitions.

Alignment is crucial to maintain during strength and flexibility exercises. Unnecessary stress may result from doing exercises poorly or in incorrect positions. If you are too tired to do the exercises correctly, do them with less intensity, do them with fewer repetitions, or do not do them at all.

Refer to the muscle chart in appendix A often. This may be useful in locating particular muscle groups you may want to target.

Upper Body

Arms and Shoulders

Often ignored by dancers, especially female dancers, strength in the upper body is crucial for the diversity of the jazz dance technique. As previously explained, the variety of movements in jazz dance today often dictate weight being carried on body parts other than the feet and legs. Be sure to strengthen any major muscle groups that will be stressed.

Arm circles (for the triceps, biceps, and deltoids, useful for port de bras)

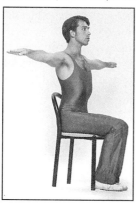 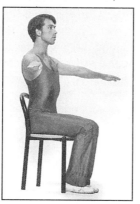 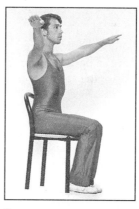 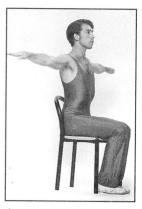

a. b. c. d.

Arm circles may either be done sitting or standing as long as the back is in proper alignment and the arms extended directly out from the shoulders. Begin with 8 slow, smooth, small circles (4–6 inches in diameter) forward and 8 backward. Repeat the set increasing the size of the circle (8–10 inches in diameter). The entire series may be done 1–8 times.

Shoulder girdle adductors[2]
Begin on the stomach in a front horizontal position, the forehead on the floor, the arms in second position. (A small pillow may be placed under the abdominals.) Rotate the entire arm until your thumbs point to the ceiling. Lift the thumbs toward the ceiling, keeping your chest and forehead on the floor. Hold for 4 counts and return to the starting position. Begin with 4 repetitions, building to 8.

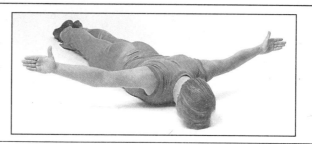

Shoulder press

Sitting in a chair with the back straight and the pelvis in a neutral position, place the hands beside the hips. Push strongly against the chair, lifting the torso up. Hold for 8 counts. Begin with 4 repetitions, building to 10.

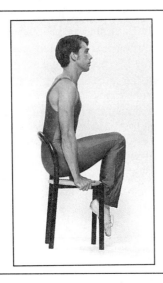

Palm press (for the pectorals and biceps, also the wrists and forearms)

It is important that the abdominals support the lower spine and that the pelvis is in a neutral position. Circle the arms from over the head, out to the sides and toward each other meeting in front of the sternum. Press the palms together firmly and hold for 10 seconds. Inhale as the arms circle and exhale as they press together. Begin with 4 repetitions, building to 8.

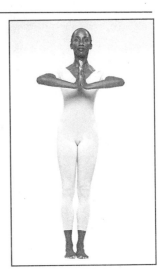

Torso

Perhaps the greatest asset to a dancer is a strong sense of "center."[3] In the strictly physical sense, center has to do with abdominal strength and providing support to the spine and pelvis. Strong abdominal muscles are crucial for maintaining proper body alignment and moving the weight through space efficiently. Judy Gantz has said that a key factor in dance injury prevention is proper movement mechanics. Well-conditioned torso muscles are integral to proper movement.[4] In particular for abdominal strength, the dancer should do exercises to increase the strength and endurance of the transversus abdominus and internal obliques. (See muscle chart, appendix A.)

Pelvic tilts

Inhale while the lower back releases and slightly arches, exhale as the lumbar spine reaches to the floor, the abdominals contract and hollow, and the bottom of the pelvis tilts upward. The feet are flat on the floor, the legs parallel, and the knees bent. The arms remain relaxed on the floor beside the body. For strength and endurance, build from 1 set of 10 repetitions to 4 sets.

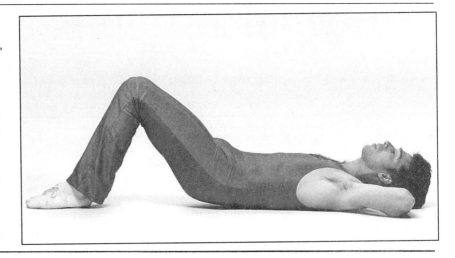

Roll downs (for the transversus abdominus, internal obliques, external obliques, and rectus abdominus)

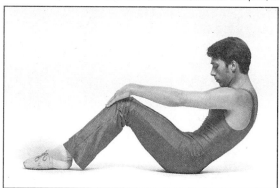

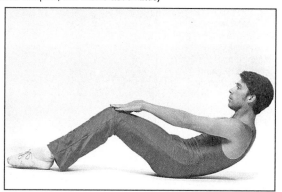

a. With the feet flat on the floor, and the knees bent close to the buttocks, begin by contracting and exhaling. Roll down slowly through the spine as if lowering one vertebra at a time.

b. Take 8 counts to lower and 8 counts to return to sitting. Lower only until the bottom of the shoulder blades touch the floor, and only raise to the contracted beginning position. Begin with 4 repetitions, increasing to 10 as strength builds.

Roll downs (for the internal obliques)

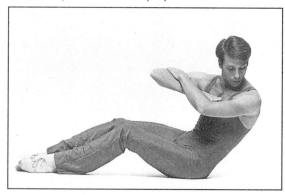

a.

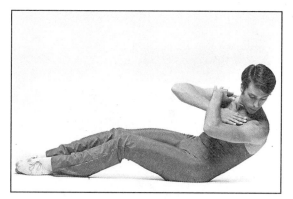

b.

Roll downs may be done lowering to the left side with the weight over the left hip and looking to the left. Repeat on the right. Always keep a concave shape, with the abdominals flat and contracted. Remember to exhale deeply at the beginning of each roll and to keep the abdominals working on the inhalation. Begin with 4 repetitions, increasing to 10 as strength builds.

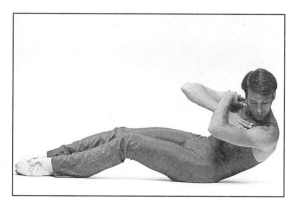

c.

Increasing the intensity of the roll down

To increase the resistance and the difficulty of the exercise, cross the arms in front of the body, or place a 5-pound weight on the chest.

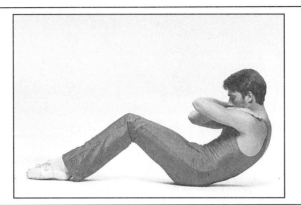

The following exercise is a great toner. The motion of pulling the knee down to the chest stretches the lower back and hamstrings; the reach contracts the lower and upper abdominal muscles, and it stretches the muscles of the neck and shoulders.

Single leg stretches[5]

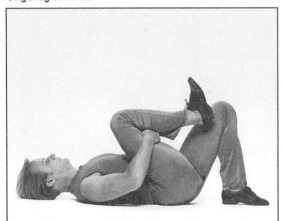

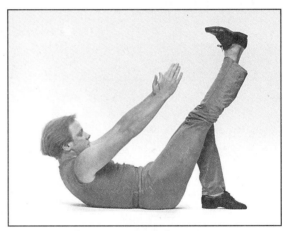

a. Start in the same position as the pelvic tilts. Draw the right knee toward the chest, being sure to grab behind the knee as you inhale deeply. Keep the foot flexed at all times, the hips as square as possible.

b. Lift the head, contract the abdominal muscles, and exhale. As you exhale, extend your leg until it is straight and parallel with the thigh of the bent leg. At the same time, extend your arms parallel to the stretched leg, keeping the lower back pressed to the floor. Begin with 4 repetitions, increasing to 10 as strength builds.

Lower Body

Turnout

As mentioned in chapter 2, turnout, or outward rotation of the legs at the hip, is a personal action, different on each dancer's body. Factors contributing to the degree of turnout are the length of ligaments and tendons, the flexibility of muscles in this area, and bone structure. The dancer may strengthen his/her turnout with the following exercises.

Spirals/Crosses/"v's" (for the adductors of the inner thigh, biceps femoris, and sartorius.
As these exercises are for rotation and not for developing abdominal strength, the hands may be placed under the hips, palms down, if necessary.)

Spirals

Lying on the back with the feet extended directly toward the ceiling, flex the feet. From a parallel position, spiral the legs to an outward rotation, initiating the action with the muscles around the top of the thigh. Try to keep the heels close together as you continue for 4 counts. Rotate back to parallel and repeat the exercise 4 times to start, increasing to 10 times as strength builds.

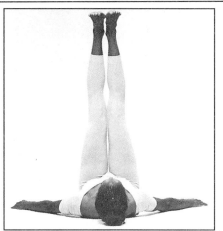

a.

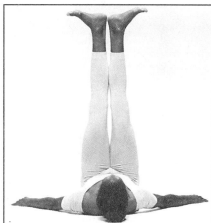

b.

Crosses

In the same position, turn out the legs and cross one in front of the other toe to heel. Continue to spiral from the top of the thighs as you alternate crosses, first right in front then left. Cross 8 times, bend the knees to rest the legs, then repeat. Eventually build to 4 sets of 8, then increase the repetitions to 16 and build to 4 sets.

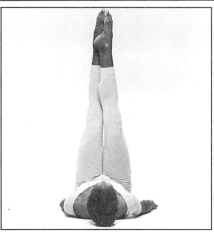

a.

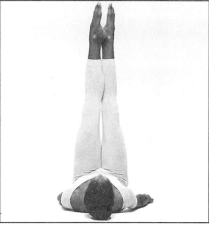

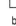

b.

Thighs

The second exercise on the following page works the knee and hip extensors and is useful for running and jumping. Make sure the thigh does not pass the 90-degree mark as this will unnecessarily stretch the ligaments in the front of the knee.

Ankles and Feet

The exercise on page 61 will serve the dancer well in developing both strength and flexibility in the ankles, feet, and lower legs for jumping and for being in the relevé position. It is extremely important to maintain the correct alignment with each execution.

Vs

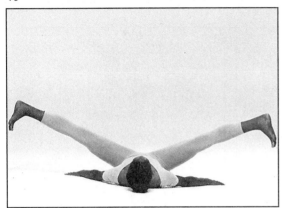

a.

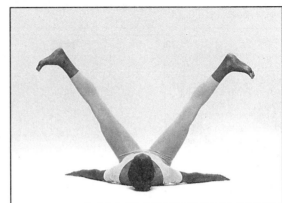

b.

Also in the same position, open the legs as wide as possible, continuing to spiral them outward. Take 16 slow counts to bring the heels together, keeping the legs extended. Build to 4 repetitions. As in all the exercises, visualizing the muscles of the hip and legs spiraling outward as you are doing the action will complement the work (see chapter 1—Visualization).

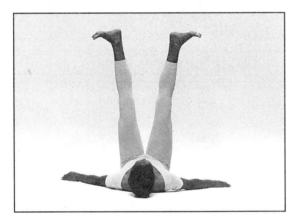

c.

Lunges (for the quadriceps and hamstrings) Begin by checking your alignment. Take a large step forward and bend the forward leg. Your knee should not be farther forward than the toes. Push yourself back up to the starting position and repeat with other leg. Repeat this set 4 times to start, building to 8 sets.

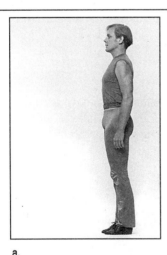

a.

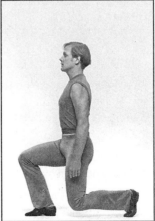

b.

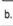

Heel raises (for the gastrocnemius, soleus [calf muscles], tibialis anterior [front of the lower leg], ankles, and feet)

a. Begin by standing with the toes and balls of the feet on the edge of a stair or other level, elevated surface. Be sure that the feet are close together (no more than a couple of inches apart) and *absolutely parallel*, the abdominals are supporting the lower spine, and the spine is in good alignment. Placing a hand on the nearby wall for balance is recommended. Lower the heels below the stair gently and slowly, hold for a minimum of 8 counts, retaining proper alignment.

b. Rise slowly to the relevé position, then repeat. Start with 4 repetitions, building to 2 sets of 10 repetitions each. Deceptively difficult, this exercise will strengthen the lower leg and feet and stretch the muscles of the calf and the attachment to the Achilles tendon.

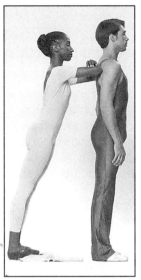 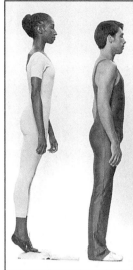

a.   b.

Variation on heel raises

a. A variation of this exercise begins the same way, with similar emphasis on correct alignment. From the relevé position this time, lower the right heel below the stair, while flexing the left knee. Allow most of the weight to be borne on the right leg, without distorting the alignment of the hips and spine.

b. Rise to relevé on both feet again and repeat with the left heel. Alternate feet building to 2 sets of 10 repetitions.

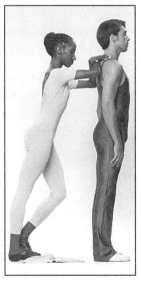 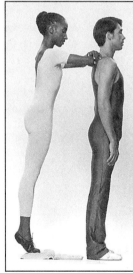

a.   b.

Summary

Balanced strength and flexibility in as many areas of the body as possible is the goal of supplemental training. Often when strength and flexibility increase, so do one's muscular control and coordination.

There is a difference between *muscular strength*, which is the ability of the muscles to generate maximum force against resistance, and *muscular*

Checklist: Strength Training

- Variety in any training program is necessary to achieve progress.
- Using the muscle chart in Appendix A will help you identify and locate the muscles you will be targeting.
- Using the visualization techniques described in chapter 1 will complement this work.
- Injured dancers, or those with structural or alignment difficulties, should first seek the counsel of a physician or other professional who can give them **personal attention and advice**.
- There is a **special relationship** between strength and flexibility that dictates that opposing muscle groups be balanced in strength and flexibility to allow the fullest movement.
- **Overloading** is the concept that the stress must continually be increased for the capacity of the body to increase.
- **Repetitions** are the number of exercises done in each set.
- It is important to always maintain proper **alignment**.

endurance, which is the ability of the muscle to contract over a continued period of time. To increase strength, the muscles will have to be worked progressively harder, increasing the resistance or the frequency of the work. To increase their endurance, the muscles will have to be worked for longer durations.

Remember that the best way to learn how to dance, however, is to dance; these exercises cannot take the place of the formal, careful instruction of a good jazz class. If not taking a class, the dancer should do a personal warm-up before the strength training (see chapter 1) and finish with a cool-down.

Endnotes

1. If the exercises are not done in conjunction with dance class, it is advantageous to design a workout that will include a personal warm-up, strength conditioning for all the major muscle groups, some endurance activity, flexibility exercises for all the major muscle groups used, and a cool-down. This type of program could be done 3 times a week. Pay attention to all the training concepts listed in this chapter, such as overloading and repetitions, to get the most out of each session.
2. Adapted from: P. Clarkson and A. Watkins, *Dancing Longer, Dancing Stronger* (Princeton, N.J.: Dance Horizons/Princeton Book Co., Pub., 1990), 233–34.
3. Please see chapter 1 for more on "center."
4. See Judy Gantz, "Dance Technique: Understanding the Contraction," *Dance Teacher Now*, September 1987, 31–36.
5. Adopted from: Benno Isaacs and Jay Kobler, *The Nicklaus Technique* (New York: A&W Publishers, Inc., 1978).

CHAPTER 6

Supplemental Flexibility Training for the Dancer

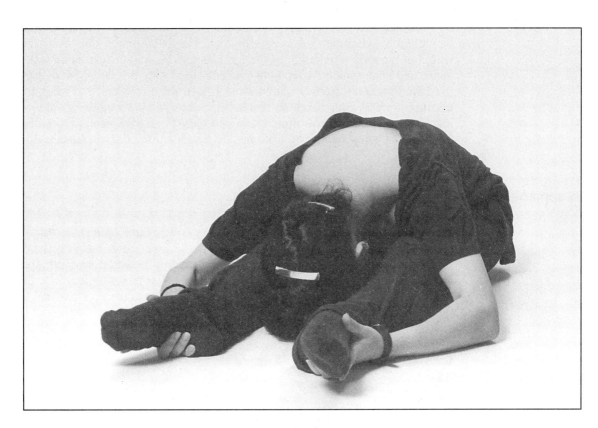

Outline

Balanced strength and flexibility in as many parts of the body as possible is the goal of supplemental training. This chapter has a few suggestions of exercises that when done properly will help improve the dancer's flexibility in some areas.

You will recall from the last chapter that variety in any training program is necessary to achieve progress. If the dancer is not taking a class, he/she should first do a personal warm-up [see chapter 1] and finish with a cool-down. Using the muscle chart in appendix A will help you identify which muscles you will be targeting and where they are. The visualization techniques described in chapter 1 will complement the work.

Flexibility is a personal accomplishment, and your range of motion cannot be judged by what you see in other bodies. Flexibility is determined by the length of muscles, the length of the tendons and ligaments surrounding the joints, and bone structure. As no two bodies are exactly the same, the degree to which they can stretch certain muscle groups will also differ. You will want to concentrate on your own body and become absorbed in recognizing the feeling of safe stretching. You should be able to feel the tight muscles loosening gradually as you stretch, but avoid feeling a sudden pull or pain close to the joints.

Supplemental Flexibility Training

Flexibility is defined as the range of motion possible at the joints, ascertained by the elongation and lengthening of muscle fibers. Some muscles have to contract for others to lengthen, providing **the relationship between strength and flexibility**. Most dancers strive for and most dance disciplines demand a great deal of flexibility in the legs and torso. It may take years to develop this kind of flexibility, and it should be done thoughtfully and carefully. Proper alignment is essential as it creates the least amount of stress on the body while allowing optimum stretch. Stretching correctly and within your *personal* anatomical limitations may also help prevent some injuries.[1]

Warm-up

The following are some points to consider when stretching. Warm-up is absolutely necessary *before* stretching. Review chapter 1 and remember to raise the body temperature one to two degrees. Being warm will enable the muscles to be more pliable and conducive to the stretch. The most effective stretching may actually be done after class when the body has had a thorough workout.

Relaxation

Though there are several different methods of stretching,[2] relaxation and breathing are common keys to stretching effectively (again review chapter 1). The body is equipped with an automatic protection system called the "stretch reflex": Muscles will actually *contract* to prevent injury or trauma in response to ballistic or sudden stresses. Obviously this is an opposite action than desired. Slow, sustained stretches allow the muscle to elongate gradually, bypassing the stretch reflex. Breathing deeply can also aid in this process. The body tends to relax more easily with an exhalation. (As an illustration, gasp, as if startled, and notice the body's natural response: to inhale and tighten up; now sigh as if exhausted and notice how the body relaxes with the exhale.) A very effective stretching method is to remain calm, not moving on the inhale, and to stretch carefully and slowly on the exhale, using full connected breaths.

Duration

The length of time you stretch each muscle group, or the duration of the stretch, must be long enough for the muscle to relax and elongate. If you isolate the stretch to the belly of the muscle, you will be able to feel when the tension begins to release. If you are very warm and flexible to begin with, thirty to ninety seconds in each area several times a week may be sufficient. The dancer with tighter muscles may want to increase this to as long as several minutes in each area five or six times a week. Like any training program, the exercises must be varied for there to be gain in flexibility.

Specificity

Take another look at the muscle chart to locate the groups you wish to work. Effective stretching mandates that you be specific in your approach, taking care to isolate the stretch to the belly of the muscle where the elongation capacity is approximately one and a half times its resting state. *Muscles* are the only fibers that can stretch safely. They are pliable and elastic and will return to their resting state with little trauma. *Tendons*, on the other hand, attach muscle to bone, and while they are pliable, tendons are not elastic. As with *ligaments*, which attach bone to bone, tendons do not contract. When stretched, they will not return to their normal length. If you feel a stretching sensation close to, or in, the joint, adjust your body so the sensation is in the large, middle section of the muscle. Isolating the proper area will become easier as you become more in tune with your body. Be sure to use the visualization techniques.

Remember that this is your body, and stretching is a personal accomplishment not to be judged by the anatomy and capabilities of others. (Please see chapter 3 for stretching within the class framework.)

Upper Body

Shoulders (trapezius, deltoids, pectoralis major)

You can easily stretch the muscles of the shoulders, upper back and chest with the following exaggerated shoulder circles. Sit in a chair with the spine erect and pressing against the back of the chair.

Torso

One of the safest ways to stretch the back is illustrated below. This method protects and supports the lower spine. Using the abdominals to support the lumbar region is suggested for all stretches.

Make sure to also do stretches for the hip flexors (quadriceps, iliopsoas, and adductor groups) and the extensors (hamstrings, gluteus medius, and gluteus maximus) so they do not pull on the pelvic girdle, altering the alignment of the lower back.

Exaggerated Shoulder Circles

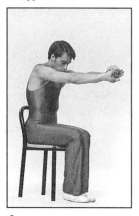 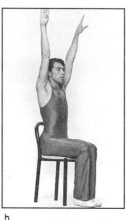 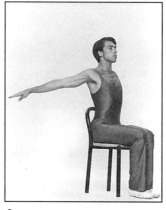 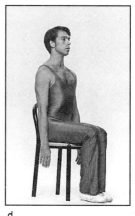

a.   b.   c.   d.

Clasp the hands in front of the body and reach as far forward as possible, rounding the shoulders. Keep the spine pressed to the chair and reach up, lifting the shoulders as high as possible. Now unclasp the hands and reach behind the chair, keeping the out-stretched arms at shoulder level. Finally, drop the arms to the sides and reach as far down as possible, taking care not to distort the alignment of the spine. Be sure to keep the abdominal muscles working, supporting the lower back and preventing any hyper-extension of the lumbar region.

The exercise may also be done without the chair. Make sure the spine is in correct alignment to begin and remains erect as the stretch occurs. With each reach exhale deeply and count to 4. Return to the starting position on the inhale. Two complete sets to start will be sufficient. Increase to 6 as needed.

Curled position

Make sure that the top of the head is on the floor. Hold this position until you feel the lower back release. Keep breathing deeply.

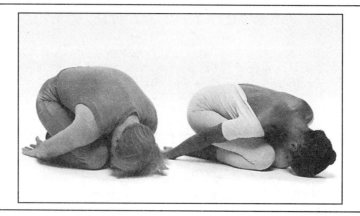

Lower Body

Turnout

These stretches concentrate on the adductors of the inner thigh and the gluteus groups. An additional stretch for the inner thighs is on page 37.

Tailor sit or gluteal stretch

With the legs either crossed as in a tailor sit or one over the other, inhale as you feel the abdominals lifted and the spine erect. Exhale, and relax the body over the legs to feel a stretch in the gluteus medius and gluteus maximus. Stay in this position for 4 or 5 continuous circular breaths. You will also feel the stretch in the hip abductors and tensor fascia lata. Keep the abdominals working. Return to the beginning position and repeat.

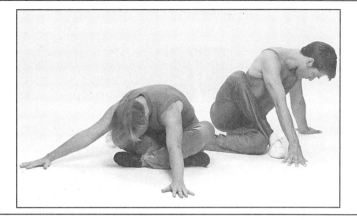

Hamstring stretch

Exhale as you lower the chest to the thigh, and make sure that the chest remains on the thigh throughout to protect the lower back.[3] Keep breathing for at least 30–90 seconds. As the hamstring relaxes, gently straighten the leg. If more of a stretch is needed, flex the foot. Engage the abdominals strongly to lift the back up to standing. Repeat as often as needed on both legs.

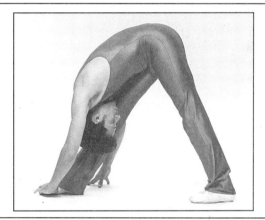

Thighs

Quadricep stretch

While holding on to a wall, reach the right hand back to the toe of the right foot. Try not to squish the knee but rather pull the abdominals up away from the thigh. Stretch the front of the thigh for 30–90 seconds. Release and repeat on the other leg. Repeat the entire set as needed.

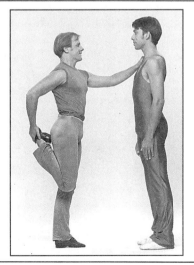

Ankles and Feet

Checklist: Supplemental Flexibility Training

- Flexibility is defined as the range of motion possible at the joints.
- Flexibility is determined by the length of muscles, the length of the tendons and ligaments surrounding the joints, and bone structure.
- Warm-up is absolutely necessary *before* stretching.
- Relaxation and breathing are keys to stretching effectively.

Summary

When determining a flexibility-enhancing program for yourself remember to keep in mind the checkpoints listed above. Listen to your own body, become in-tune with its idiosyncracies and limitations and do not judge yourself against others. Also, be sure to use all you've learned about warm-up, relaxation, and visualization.

Endnotes

1. Coaches Roundtable. "Prevention of Athletic Injuries through Strength Training and Conditioning," *National Strength and Conditioning Association Journal*, vol. 5, no. 2, 14–19.
2. For good discussions on methods of stretching see:
   Gigi Berardi, *Finding Balance: Fitness and Training for a Lifetime in Dance* (Princeton, N.J.: Dance Horizons/Princeton Book Co., Pub., 1991).
   Martha Myers, "Facts and Fantasies: Stretching," *Dance Magazine*, June 1990, 66–70.
   Coaches Roundtable. "Flexibility," *National Strength and Conditioning Association Journal*, vol. 6, no. 4, 10–22.
   S.P. Sady, "Flexibility Training: Ballistic, Static, or Proprioceptive Neuromuscular Facilitation?" *Archives of Physical Medicine Rehabilitation* 63:261–63.
3. J. Alter, *Surviving Exercise* (Boston: Houghton Mifflin Co., 1983). She explains that the lower back is jeopardized when doing an unsupported stretch. Keeping the chest on the thigh whether the knee is flexed or elongated will help lessen this hazard.

CHAPTER 7

Discipline and Training Schedules

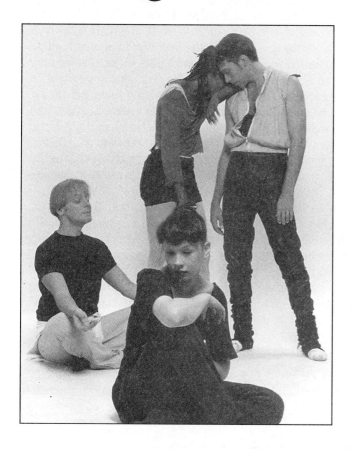

Outline

Discipline and Training Schedule
Checklist: A Positive Mental Attitude
Variety in Training
Body Therapies
Scheduling
Summary

Discipline and Training Schedules

When developing a training schedule it is important to consider the capabilities and limitations of the human body. In an effort to achieve near perfection or virtuosity (the leg must always be higher, the leaps have more amplitude), dancers often have the tendency to overtrain, misuse and even abuse their instruments.

Though it is true that most serious dancers need to train five or six days a week and that basic exercises have to be repeated often to accomplish flawlessness, it is also true that alternating routines is the best way to prevent fatigue and overuse. It is important to recover between workouts.[1] Rest is absolutely essential for developing muscles to allow time for the fuels that are expended during exercise to be replaced. (In general, strength-building regimens should be done every other day, while endurance activities, which metabolize fat stores for energy, could be done each day.) Remember to keep in mind your dance goals and devise a program to fit your individual needs. In the beginning, dancing two to three times a week may be sufficient, increasing training only as the knowledge of technique, body mechanics, strength, and personal capability increases.

Discipline in sticking to your training, and discipline in training your mind are equally important factors. Throughout this book there have been many suggestions for using intellectual, physical and emotional processes to achieve success. We suggest reviewing the sections devoted to mental preparation, including visualization and relaxation techniques (chapter 1), and the "Checklist on Preparing for a Successful Class" (chapter 3) often. It is very important to reexamine these chapters soon after your first classes, as the experiences will help further your understanding of the methodology. A positive attitude, concentration, and relaxation should not be overlooked as vital aspects of any training schedule, and the best time to initiate mental training is at the beginning of participation in any dance form or program.

Checklist: A Positive Mental Attitude

- Inhale and exhale fully, prompting yourself to be relaxed.
- Free yourself of tension, eliminate any stressful thoughts, and concentrate fully on the class to come.
- Begin warm-ups slowly, allowing time to adjust to vigorous movement.
- Develop your levels of concentration and stamina slowly and consistently.
- Watch the teacher carefully during the demonstrations.
- Use external visualization to imagine yourself doing the exercises as if on TV.
- Imagine how the muscles would feel if they were doing the exercise.
- Do not feel pressured to push yourself to a level beyond your capability.
- Concentrate on your own dancing.
- Do the best you can and enjoy it.

Variety in Training

Rather than taxing the muscles by repeating the same routine each day, the serious dancer should consider *variety* in training. While many professional jazz dancers also take ballet classes, there are many other dance forms to explore, such as tap, flamenco, modern, or ballroom dancing. (The latter can be very helpful in providing the training needed for eventual partnering or for shows on Broadway, if that is a goal.) You could also vary your training by studying with teachers who emphasize largely different aspects of the jazz technique. This will have you moving in different ways, both modifying and contrasting exercises. You can also interject your program with aerobic and weight training.

Variety will help to prevent burnout, which may be brought on by persistent allegiance to goals that you have set for yourself. Enthusiasm and energy are a part of all dance forms, and keeping up your motivation is important. If you experience mental, physical, or emotional exhaustion, change your schedule somewhat, review the relaxation techniques, or lighten up for a while. Motor learning research has shown that more is not always better in regard to training sessions, and time off can sometimes help to invigorate and rejuvenate the dancer/athlete.[2]

Body Therapies

In addition, many dancers find body therapies and reeducation programs such as the Alexander Technique, Bartinieff Fundamentals, the Pilates Method, Ideokinesis, or Feldenkrais beneficial.[3] Body therapies tend to use the brain and passive methods to repattern faulty technique and reduce tension and stress in movement. Many help to prevent injuries by increasing overall awareness of motion and expressiveness. They re-educate by directing the dancer's attention to habitual movement patterns as a prelude to changing those that are inefficient, limiting, or harmful. The body therapies have in common the goal of altering the way muscles pattern themselves.[4] Using a mind-body connection, they help the dancer modify movement and maintain health.

Alexander Technique

Many think that the Alexander Technique must be experienced to be understood as it is often referred to as learning how to "not do" rather than do, or to "inhibit" moving in an incorrect manner.[5] The aim of the technique is to distribute stresses and tension evenly throughout the entire body. Frederick Matthias Alexander (1869–1955) deduced that through *Primary Control* (the balanced relationship of the head to the body that produces the least amount of tension in the neck),[6] moving with less effort could be achieved. Students learn this in a practical way through the gentle guiding of a teacher's hands. The first objective is to learn how the freedom of the neck and poise of the head are essential to a coordinated, light, balanced state. The exercises include "relearning" how to do everyday movements such as walking, standing from and sitting into a chair, lifting the arms, etc. The results are awareness of one's movement habits and re-education of the body to eliminate or prevent inefficient habits from reoccurring. Alexander asserted that relaxation in action can produce an ease and economy of movement, an efficiency that is the direct aim of every dancer. The American Center for the Alexander Technique, Inc., is located at 129 West 67th Street, New York, NY 10023 (212-799-0468). Here one can get information on teacher training, referrals, and a list of the Alexander centers.

Bartinieff Fundamentals

Irmgard Bartinieff founded the Laban/Bartinieff Institute of Movement Studies in 1978 and continued to explore, explain, and develop the theories of Rudolph Laban, the inventor of Labananalysis or Laban Movement Studies. Laban and his colleagues devised a method of analyzing movement for both its functional and expressive implications.[7] Using this analysis, Bartinieff developed the Fundamentals. These exercises are designed to reawaken one's awareness of muscles and joints that are not used, are used inadequately, or are misused. The objective is to extend movement potential in both energy and expressiveness, as well as extend the range of movement. The basic exercises always stress the diagonal connections between the top and lower parts of the body and the relationship to the entire spine. The first six floor exercises are simple lifting, lowering, flexing and extending limbs or body parts with the concentration on articulation and physiological changes. The Fundamentals are explained and illustrated in Bartinieff's *Body Movement: Coping with the Environment*. The Laban/Bartinieff Institute of Movement Studies, Inc., is located at 31 West 27th Street, New York, NY 10001 (212-689-0740).

Pilates® Method

Joseph Pilates believed in physical and mental harmony and brought his method of conditioning to the United States in the early 1920s. The exercises are done both on the floor and aboard a *reformer*, an apparatus whose carriage slides back and forth upon a frame, outfitted with springs, and straps. The springs provide a graduated tension for exercises that have direct application to the movements of athletes and dancers, such as relevés and pliés. The series of precise movements promotes sleekness of muscle tone instead of bulk. Without the stress of gravity, and with the guided direction of a Pilates instructor, participants may increase strength and flexibility, rehabilitate injuries, and fix faulty technique habits. The role of the abdominals and lower back muscles is stressed in most exercises, and this area becomes the "powerhouse of the body."[8] True balance and total coordination of mind and body are emphasized.[9] Pilates students must concentrate fully on exact alignment, executing every repetition correctly. Results of this method have proved in many cases to be quite remarkable. Many famous dancers such as Martha Graham, George Balanchine, members of the American Ballet Theatre, and Jerome Robbins have used Pilates, in addition to athletes such as Martina Navratilova, Chris Evert, and Kristy Yamaguchi. Romana Kryzanowska was chosen by Joseph Pilates to carry on the tradition of his unique method. She is associated with the Pilates Studio in New York City, located at 2121 Broadway, 10023 (800-223-7691). The Institute for the Pilates® Method is located in Santa Fe, New Mexico (505-988-1990).

Ideokinesis

In her book *The Thinking Body*, Mabel Todd said that "imagination itself, or the inner image, is a form of physical expression, and the motor response is the reflection of it."[10] She also noted, "Changing the attitudes of the body is one way to change the mental attitudes; conversely, changing the mental attitudes certainly changes the bodily."[11] With these theories and an intense study into the power of mental and physiological processes on all physical movements, Todd provided a new means of dealing with movement that would use the power of imagination. Building on these treatises, Dr. Lulu Sweigard created a comprehensive body of material called *Ideokinesis*, (from ideo meaning idea and kinesis meaning physical movement). This method of re-educating is founded in guided visualization as a tool for changing movement and movement patterns. Sweigard felt that if one concentrated on the image of a movement, the body itself would find the most efficient and noninjurious way of achieving it. An exercise in this method may ask the student to lie on his/her back, with the knees pointed toward the ceiling and the feet as close to the buttocks as possible, and imagine sand pouring through the thigh into the pelvis and out the back onto the floor. The image is a means of releasing tension in the quadriceps and lengthening the lumbar region of the spine. Visualization as a learning technique is stressed; imagining, pretending, and watching are often used as directives. Sweigard also stressed balanced skeletal alignment as a basis for all efficient movement. Irene Dowd, most notably, has continued on with Todd/Sweigard's theories of Ideokinesis, functional anatomy, and neuromuscular re-education. She has maintained a private practice out of New York City for the past 20 years.[12]

Feldenkrais

Like the other body therapies, Moshe Feldenkrais developed a re-education system based on the correction of faulty movement patterns, ease of movement, and freedom of breath. His technique stresses sensing and making accurate assessments of one's own body and body parts. It may be done either with a certified instructor or by using the format in his book *Awareness through Movement*.[13] Feldenkrais was a learned man with a background in physics, yoga, and judo. A knee injury led him down a road of self-discovery and education bringing anatomy, physiology, and learning theories together in the healing process. He founded the Feldenkrais Institute in Tel Aviv, Israel, and today certified instructors teach his technique throughout the world. The Feldenkrais method uses early childhood coordinations, organic breathing patterns, and attention to a more articulate spine in exercises that may be as simple as a head moving back and forth, or rolling over on the floor. Low-grade, repetitive motion is characteristic of this approach.[14]

Massage

In the past, the art of massage suffered an unfortunate, poor public image due mainly to disreputable massage parlors. Now gaining more respect, massage and massage therapies have proved beneficial for dancers and athletes as a method of relieving tension and muscle soreness and increasing the range of movement. Massage may also help to control fatigue and increase endurance by dispersing accumulated fatigue products (lactic acid) that can irritate the muscles after exercise.[15] To eliminate this irritation, masseurs seek to stimulate the metabolic process, thereby hastening reabsorption and release rates of wastes. Massage can help break down scar tissue and increase blood circulation, both relieving pain and accelerating the healing process, and on its most basic level is therapeutic just because of its pleasurable experience.[16] It is no wonder that massage therapies are popular among athletes and dancers and can be rejuvenating, healthy experiences.

Scheduling

Economics, intensity of training, professional goals, and other factors will influence your training schedule, and it is best not to get distressed trying to fit everything into your life. If life were perfect, however, the dancer serious about pursuing a career may choose to take five or six dance classes per week. (A professional dancer takes some form of dance class, does some other type of training, and has several hours of rehearsals five or six days a week.) In addition, two or three low to moderate intensity endurance work-outs, one or two strength/flexibility work-outs and a weekly massage would contribute greatly to his/her overall physical condition. (Remember that endurance workouts can be done every day, while strength workouts should have a minimum of twenty-four hours in between. An ideal schedule may look like the following:

Mon.	Tues.	Wed.	Thurs.	Fri.	Sat.	Sun.
Jazz Dance	Ballet	Jazz Dance	Ballet	Jazz Dance	Jazz Dance	Off
Body therapy	Aerobics (Ex:walking biking, or swimming	Strength/ Flexibility (Ex: Yoga, or Pilates)	Aerobics (Or tap dance, ballroom or modern	Strength/ Flexibility workout	Massage	Off

This would truly be an ideal schedule for the serious dancer. As a typical jazz dance class is often slightly more aerobic than a ballet class, we have grouped workouts in the above fashion. Following this schedule a dancer would be doing endurance and technique training every day, beginning each week with a body therapy, and rewarding themselves with a massage at the end of the week. When designing your schedule be sensible and don't overdo it. Fatigue is one of the major causes of injuries and is unnecessary.

If you experience headaches, shakiness, an increase in nervousness, excess soreness, or a desire to quit,[17] slow down. There is no good reason to push yourself into an emotional or physical state of exhaustion. Overtraining the mind and body can only cause burnout and will not help to improve your overall mental or dance fitness.

Whichever you choose, and however you arrange your schedule, remember that only technically correct repetition will provide a continual basis for improvement. The dancer needs a thoughtful teacher and observer to monitor placement and movement and a variety of exercises to provide a balance of flexibility and strength to as many areas of the body as possible.

Summary

The art of dance is a complex and intriguing form that requires a mind-body-spirit connection. It utilizes processes in the physical, intellectual and emotional realms. It is an art of communication that has many layers. Studying dance demands attention to all of these areas. To give yourself the best chance adopt a positive working attitude and follow sensible nutritional practices. Supplement your training with an endurance, strength, and flexibility component if necessary, and devise a disciplined training schedule. Be sure to include variety and have fun. Enjoying your training will be the best insurance of sticking to it.

Endnotes

1. Dr. Hans Selye demonstrated that if rats were stressed and allowed to recover, they became stronger. If they were stressed again before they recovered, they became weaker. From:
   Hans, Selye, *Stress without Distress* (New York: Lippincott and Crowell Publishers, 1974).
2. Keith P. Henschen, "Athletic Staleness and Burnout: Diagnosis, Prevention and Treatment," *Applied Sports Psychology* (Mountain View, Calif.: Mayfield Pub., 1986), 327–41.
3. For more on body therapies see:
   Martha Myers and Margaret Pierpont, "Body Therapies and the Modern Dancer," *Dance Magazine.* August 1983 (Special Pullout Section).
4. Martha Myers, "Body Therapies and the Modern Dancer: The New Science of Dance Training," *Dance Magazine*, February 1980, 90–92.
5. Frank Ottiwell, "The Alexander Technique: A Matter of Choice" *Your Body Works: A Guide to Health, Energy and Balance,* ed. Gerald Kogan (Berkeley, Calif.: And/Or Transformations Press, 1980).
6. Ottiwell, 67.
7. Irmgard Bartinieff with Dori Lewis, *Body Movement: Coping with the Environment* (New York: Gordon and Breach Science Pub., 1980).
8. From a private conversation with Anthony Rabarra, Certified Pilates instructor, Princeton, N.J.
9. Philip Friedman and Gail Eisen, *The Pilates Method of Physical and Mental Conditioning* (New York: Warner Books, Inc., 1980).
10. Mabel E. Todd, *The Thinking Body* (Princeton, N.J.: A Dance Horizons Book/Princeton Book Company, 1968).
11. Todd, 295.
12. For further reading see: Irene Dowd, *Taking Root to Fly: ten articles on functional anatomy* (New York: Contact Editions, Irene Dowd, 1990).
13. Moshe Feldenkrais, *Awareness through Movement* (New York: Harper & Row Publishers, 1972).
14. Sally Sevey Fitt, *Dance Kinesiology* (New York: Schirmer Books, 1988).

15. Gordon Inkeles, *The New Massage* (New York: A Perigee Book/G.P. Putnam's Sons, 1980).

16. For more on massage see:
Daniel Nagrin, *How to Dance Forever: Surviving against the Odds* (New York: William Morrow and Co., Inc., 1988), 141–43.

17. Steven J. Fleck and William J. Kraemer, "The Overtraining Syndrome," *National Strength and Conditioning Association Journal*, September 1982, 50–51.

CHAPTER 8

What Is Jazz Dance?

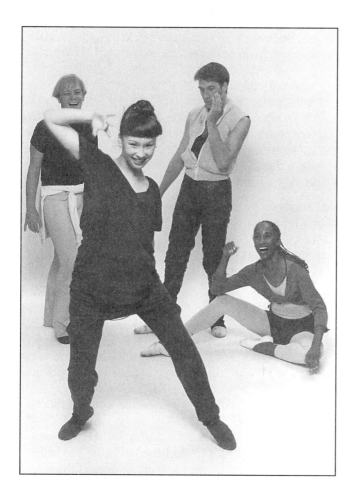

Outline

America's Folk Dance

"America's folk dance"—that's what Jack Cole, an early jazz giant, called jazz dance in an oft-quoted description. It reflects America: the energy and lethargy, the naiveté and cruelty, the confidence and insecurity, the good and bad.

Jazz dance is everywhere, like some kind of cultural fog: in the streets, in the clubs, on stages, and on television; it's in university classrooms, on MTV, and in strip-joints. It's difficult to grab on to this jazz-fog as it constantly changes before our eyes, shifting quickly from the sublime to the vulgar to the joyous.

So what is jazz dance? What makes jazz dance jazz? And is it respectable? Is it relevant? Is it art? Those of us who do it, know it's a fun and worthwhile activity; but for the serious student of jazz dance, teachers, and scholars, these questions, and more, must be conscientiously addressed. Before one embarks on a career in jazz dance or even indulges in what is a time-consuming and disciplined hobby, one would do well to consider its value to our lives and culture.

- Is jazz dance a serious art form?
- Is art an idealization or a reflection of a culture?
- Is art, by definition, upper class and aristocratic?
- Is jazz dance really an American art form?

It is in the study of jazz dance that we come face to face with issues such as these, and we will address them in this chapter as we create a portrait of jazz dance today.

We asked some successful jazz dancers, dance teachers, and choreographers for help in this task. These dance masters had a clear and confident vision of what jazz dance is . . . perhaps that's why they are masters. The checklist on page 79 summarizes the most popular definitions of jazz dance while highlighting the importance, the necessity, of individual variation and vision.

Though there are some delightful variations of emphasis in our experts' descriptions, we found in these and other interviews one singular point of common reference: all refer to the close and unique relationship between the music and the dance. The excitement, the challenge, and the beauty of the art are found in the often very complex interchange between the rhythm of the music and the rhythm of the dance. Jazz moves. Jazz swings!

Jazz Energy: The Kinetic Push

The relationship of music and dance breeds energy: this is the defining characteristic of jazz. In dance, the impulse to move is called kinetic energy. In today's jazz dance, kinetic energy comes mostly from the music. It's not surprising that this music moves us as it does. As Dizzy Gillespie once said, "Jazz music was invented for people to dance to."[1]

Energy is embedded in the soul of jazz and in the soul of its descendants and offshoots (rock and roll, pop, rap). It's built into the structure of jazz music: in its slouching melodic scale, its wailing instrumentation, and its syncopation. Leonard Bernstein emphasizes the physicality of syncopation in the following explanation:

"A good way to understand syncopation might be to think of a heart-
beat that goes along steadily and at a moment of shock misses a

Checklist: What Experts Say

- **Lynn Simonson:** Jazz music is filled with complexities of syncopation, isolations, and rhythm. Hopefully, the jazz choreographer or teacher is inspired to create movement based on some of these same qualities.
- **Susan Stroman:** It' a form of dance that is expressive of the contemporary character. Jazz dance can be done to any music. It swings through the ages.
- **David Storey:** What makes jazz dance unique from other dance forms is the exploration of rhythm. Jazz dance, to me, is an internal reaction to the rhythm and mood of the music.
- **Danny Buraczeski:** Jazz dance is music and a strong sense of the vernacular. Both the music and the dance have strong, undeniable, and continuing roots in the vernacular.
- **Billy Siegenfeld:** I affirm the place of swing in contemporary jazz dance, even in the face of the current domination in popular music and dance consciousness by the monotonously one-rhythm sound of rock and roll. . . . [D]ancing that does not reflect the rhythmic characteristics of jazz music cannot be considered true jazz dance. . .[2]
- **Frank Hatchett:** Jazz dance is interpreting music. It's my obligation to the musician to express what he feels when he's playing. It all boils down to the relationship of the movement to the music.

beat. It is that much of a physical reaction. Technically, syncopation means either the removal of an accent where you expect one or the placing of an accent where you least expect one. In either case, there is the element of surprise and shock. The body responds to this shock either by compensating for the missing accent or by reacting to the unexpected one."[3]

Though today we most often think of dancers as responding to a beat, keeping the rhythm of a record, or following the lead of the band, this was not always the case. Music and dance were equal partners in the developing jazz art. In the early days, musicians played for the dance, and dancers were very determined about what worked for them and what didn't. In a kind of movement-based evolution, the music that survived the pre-jazz and early jazz eras was the music that fueled the dance.

"In the first half of this century, jazz musicians had dance in them when they played and jazz dancers had music in them or jazz didn't happen." (Sidney Bechet)

As we shall see, jazz came from the body. The early inventors of jazz amplified the feeling and the noises and the internal rhythms of the dancers. It was a cooperative outpouring of pent-up frustration and emotion.

This energized art developed in and for an energized culture. And still, today, the jazz culture (or context) is a participatory one, with dancers and viewers alike clapping, screaming, whooping, and moving.

Checklist: Jazz Energy

- Jazz dancers get energy from music.
- Jazz music was made for movement.
- Jazz dance classes encourage free movement, improvisation, and spontaneous responses to music.
- Jazz dancers are vocal and uninhibited in their support of fellow dancers.
- Jazz audiences, as well, are vocal and uninhibited in their responses to jazz performances.

To understand how this unique jazz energy developed, we must take a brief look at the mothers and fathers of jazz. We must witness the courage, strength, and pain of the enslaved Africans in America that eventually found a voice and a dance unique to this country.

The Jazz Culture

Considering the close relationship of jazz music and dance today, it is not surprising that what we now consider two arts were once one. In the beginning, in Africa, before jazz became jazz, there was only one art. As Portia K. Maultsby plainly states: "In the Black musical tradition, motion and music are conceptualized as one process; they do not constitute the fusion of two separate entities."[4]

This is an important point precisely because it is so different from the historical Western European way of separating music and dance, body from mind,[5] individual from group. When the unified African conceptual art met the European mind-body split, there was eventually, in America, jazz. Jazz can be said to be the product of African conceptual art being poured into a Western European mind-set in a "peculiar and penetrating"[6] culture that nourished its uniqueness.[7]

Individual Risk in a Collective Context

Generally speaking, the West African peoples lived in a collective society. Just as it was impossible for West Africans to conceive of music without dance, it was impossible for them to imagine an individual without a group. The fate of the individual and the fate of his society were very much interdependent. The survival of the society depended on strict social structures, group unity, open lines of communication, as well as individual and group strength. Cultural activities reinforced these qualities.

- Strong community ties were forged by community artmaking.
- Strong bodies developed in the days-long dance/music celebrations.
- Strong, quick minds developed in improvised rituals that often invoked trancelike altered states of consciousness.

Everyone expressed himself or herself in appropriate ways; everyone moved and shared. The culture dictated that the individual did not hold back but gave himself to the greater good of the group.

European/African Influences on American Jazz

The Africans abducted and brought to America found physical, personal, and social strength even more necessary to their survival as slaves. Music and rhythm helped them through their workday: the rhythm of work songs seemed to lighten their load. Music and dance in the slave quarters—for those slaves who were allowed them—provided the social, emotional, and physical support necessary to their courage.

But this early slave culture was repressed by a European sensibility. The seemingly strange ceremonies, loud celebrations, and uninhibited recreational dances that were held in the slave quarters were fearsome to most slave owners who had been taught by their culture and religion to stay reserved and in personal, emotional control. Fearing the power of black music, slave owners passed laws against it (the Slave Act of 1740, which banned blacks from "beating drums or blowing horns"). So, the slaves made rhythm with their feet, their hands, their mouths, their bodies.

At the same time that black music was being suppressed, many whites were teaching their slaves European hymns and popular songs and dances so that the slaves could provide them with European-style entertainment. Gradually, in this way, the rhythms, purpose, and soul of West African music dance traditions began the centuries-long fusion with the harmonies and melodic structure of European music.

Music and Movement in the Black Church

In spite of the repression of the West African music/dance art, much of its spontaneity and power survived slavery. It was in the churches of the South that African collectivism and spontaneity re-surfaced.

> "It was in the context of religion that the Negro spiritual was created—a personal and collective response to the slave experience in the United States." (Maultsby 1985, 149)

> "The religious fervor was so appealing to Blacks because they had a deeply internalized positive attitude toward outward physical expressions of spiritual zeal. . . . As a result, the Blacks . . . began to adopt Christianity in large numbers. Within this milieu, they could pursue with impunity their predilection for combining physical body motion with music in the form of rhythmical hand clapping, foot pat-

ting, head bobbing, rocking back and forth, and even dancing."
(Wilson 1985, 13–14)[8]

"The Black spiritual developed because it fulfilled the basic goal: to
integrate body movement and music." (Wilson 1985, 16)

Given this context, one can understand why the environment of today's jazz
dance class or concert is inherently different from ballet or modern. History
explains the nearly universal emphasis on moving, music, emotional release,
and collective support.

Checklist: Today's Jazz Dance Class Culture

- Jazz music and dance serve to bring people together in strength.
- Jazz dance encourages group cohesiveness.
- Jazz dance nurtures individual expression within the group activity.
- Jazz dance encourages full participation in the dance activity and
  discourages individual isolation and timidity.
- Competition in jazz dance classes is constructive and empowering,
  rather than destructive and isolating.

Social Dance/Theatrical Dance

From the birth of the spiritual in the black churches of the South, the history
of jazz music and dance follows the cultural history of the black people in
America. Work songs, gospel, ragtime, the blues, swing, rock and roll, soul, and
hip-hop all originally reflected the black experience and were later adopted by
the white culture as well.

"The Shuffle, the Slide, Snake Hips, the Funky Butt in the 10s, the Charleston and the
Black Bottom in the 20s, to the Jitterbug in the 40s—all were originally black social
dances that found their way to the stage performed either by blacks in Europe, in
vaudeville, or on the black musical circuit . . . or by white entertainers who copied
them." (Stearns 1979)

It has been said that the history of jazz is a history of black invention and
white exploitation. This was certainly true in the earliest form of stage dance.
Whites took black dance and performed it onstage *in blackface* (as in minstrel
shows) while the blacks they were imitating couldn't get jobs. Many blacks went
to Europe to perform, where they were well received. This was the experience
of Sidney Bechet, Josephine Baker, and Buddy Bradley, among others. The exo-
dus of black American jazz dancers to Europe continues to this day.

To review, what we call jazz today has an African soul, but there is also a strong European influence. The black tradition contributed, among other things, the conceptual premise of a movement and music fusion, along with the encouragement of individual expression and release, plus the power of uninhibited group support.

The white culture contributed folk and rhythmic traditions (particularly evident in the influence of Irish clog dancers), European harmonies, musical form, and disciplined training regimens, as well as paths of commercialization and, later, scholarly codification of these roots.

A brief look at the dominant dance forms of the past hundred years shows an alternating influence of black and white cultures. (For an overview of jazz dance history, please see the Jazz Dance Time Line, appendix J.)

1900–1950

- **The Teens:** Before World War I, Vernon and Irene Castle were a popular dance team. They successfully incorporated some new jazz rhythms into a refined style that the white culture could enthusiastically support. (The Castles' careers were reenacted by Fred Astaire and Ginger Rogers in the 1939 MGM musical, *The Story of Vernon and Irene Castle*.) It is interesting to note that their music arranger, Ford Dabney, was a black man who helped them to successfully adapt black rhythms for a white audience.
- **The Twenties:** The roaring Twenties began with the Harlem Renaissance, a flowering of black art and culture that brought to Broadway such musicals as *Shuffle Along* (1921) and *Runnin' Wild* (1923). The dances that were introduced in these musicals soon became universally popular jazz dances, including the national craze, the Charleston.
- **The Thirties:** The Suave Thirties saw the birth of big band jazz and the Lindy-Hop, as well as the stardom of Fred Astaire and Bill "Bojangles" Robinson. In Harlem, things weren't always suave: fierce band and dance contests (every bit as fierce as the early days of rap and street dancing in The Bronx, circa 1980) were being waged at the Savoy Ballroom and other Harlem dance halls. Downtown, predominantly white orchestras (Benny Goodman, Paul Whiteman, etc.) were playing a more commercially successful (what today we would call "crossover") jazz in clubs and on the radio.
- **The Forties:** Big band jazz, along with the jazz dance/jazz music partnership, ended with World War II and the advent of recordings. Musicians and dancers went off to war. By the end of the decade, smaller combos had superseded big bands, and records began to dominate the music industry. Jazz musicians wanted to be listened to as their music became more intricate and cerebral. Jazz dancers, meanwhile, found records to be endlessly patient while they rehearsed and "set" their dances. Jazz music and jazz dance started on two different paths, and they both began to be taken more seriously as separate arts. Choreographers like Agnes DeMille, Jack Cole, and Katherine Dunham demanded more and more from their dancers, resulting in the professionalization of Broadway and Hollywood jazz dancers. Luigi developed his jazz technique with which aspiring professional dancers developed their art.

Latin American Influences

With the 1950s, we can add an important Latin American influence to the African/European/North American jazz mélange. Latin American music swept into the ballrooms and dance studios, bringing the subtleties and intricacies of Latin rhythms to American middle-class consciousness, enriching jazz dance and music immeasurably. Leonard Bernstein (music) and Jerome Robbins (choreography) used some of these rhythms in the landmark production of *West Side Story* (1957).

West Side Story had a tremendous effect on jazz dance, raising world respect for professional jazz dancers and swelling the ranks of jazz dance classes across the country.

There could be no doubt that this jazz dance (captured and preserved on film) was an art. Brenda Bufalino, founder of the American Tap Dance Orchestra and legendary tapper, has an interesting perspective on this event and its time in jazz dance history:

> "*West Side Story* opened on Broadway in 1957. It was so good that nobody could ever top it, so jazz dance went sideways. At the same time, Honi Coles was so brilliant a tap dancer that no one could ever top him, so tap went sideways. Then rock and roll came in, subtlety went out, and everything went in another direction. . . . *West Side Story* marked the end of the classic period of jazz dance."

Since the 1950s, the history of jazz dance has become primarily a history of choreography (which is discussed in the following chapter) and a history of technical advancement. The jazz dancer became a professional who concentrated on developing technique in a safe and methodical manner, as is explained in parts 1 and 2 of this book.

Jazz Dance Today

As for jazz dance today, we seem to be on the verge of a paradigm shift. As Dan Hogan, a professional New York jazz dancer, says, "Today's jazz dancers are not even sure that what they are doing *is* jazz." In the following, we will look at some of the reasons for this confusion.

The Effect of AIDS on Jazz Dance Today

Today's dance world is reeling from the effects of a deadly epidemic. AIDS has decimated the ranks of experienced and talented jazz choreographers and dancers, as well as scholars, dance assistants, and dance partners. The result is a diminished continuity from the previous generation to the present. The experience of Susan Stroman, a Tony Award-winning choreographer, is all too typical.

> "I had a dance partner named Jeff Veazey. We danced together as a team. He was a fierce tapper. We developed a show for Equity Library Theatre called *Trading Places* about two people obsessed with old movies. Within the show Jeff and I recreated about twelve

of the famous couple dances from old movies: Fred and Ginger, Gene and Judy, etc.

"I didn't have the patience to actually sit and watch the videos—I wanted to make it up myself—but he was really exacting about the process and learned the exact steps! With his pushing me I learned so much. Jeff passed away from AIDS. I haven't performed since. I loved dancing with him. When he was gone I just had no more desire. But when I watch the different shows that I choreograph, I can see Jeff's influence up there with me. His drive and his love of the dance and his love of the theatre is up there. I can see it."

Jeff Veazey represented continuity, tradition, and scholarship in jazz dance. Stroman's astounding choreography has benefited from his creative passion. Today's jazz dance is diminished without him and so many others.

Rap and Hip-hop

The question of whether rap is jazz and whether hip-hop and street dancing are part of the jazz dance tradition is a controversial one. Though hip-hop shares many characteristics of jazz dance, there are some rather important differences that we will examine. However one feels about the style, the fact is that hip-hop is having a major influence on today's jazz dance—in classes and in the professional world.

Frank Hatchett, one of the first jazz dance teachers to incorporate hip-hop and street dance in his classes, feels that "hip-hop is a whole new thing." He cautions against using classic jazz technical standards in appreciating the dances of this new genre.

Russell Clark, a Los Angeles teacher, choreographer, and rap producer (and heir to the Clark Brothers vaudeville tap team) feels that rap music is a natural continuation of the jazz tradition and that hip-hop is speaking to contemporary problems, as did jazz to the problems of the past.

"Rap is a derivation of jazz in the sense that it is an improvisation on a theme with an interpretive aspect. Rhythmically it relates totally to African syncopation and African chant. It's chanted because you can't sustain notes when you're moving. Those choppy rhythms were created to signal people to work, to lift this rock, push that log; and, eventually, in America, to tote that barge, lift that bale.

"Rap comments—it's a reaction to slavery. All kinds of people have been enslaved. Slavery is being controlled, but where you can't be controlled is in your soul, the flight of the heart. If your body can't go, at least your heart can. This is the positive side of rap to me.

"In Los Angeles, for example, power people are living in the Hollywood Hills: a strata of controllers overlooking the people in the ghetto who are out of control. It doesn't surprise me that a rhythmic kind of work commentary or reaction would grow out of that environment.

Others, including Danny Buraczeski and Susan Stroman, agree that rap and hip-hop are another turn of the circle.

"Hip-hop is a contemporary version of the Charleston. It's a funky Charleston. There is a relationship, a specific link." (Buraczeski 1992)

"It's a definite form of jazz dance, of course. It's derivative. All that popping is what Gwen Verdon was doing eighteen years ago in *Chicago*. It's Bob Fosse. Hip-hop has grown from jazz dance and will probably go back as all things do revolve back." (Stroman 1992)

Max Roach, the jazz drummer, thinks that "rap music is incredibly relevant. The young rappers today are like Charlie Parker, or even more like Louis Armstrong, true originals, because they are inventing a whole new language."

Rob Gibson, director of Jazz at Lincoln Center, is unambiguous: "Since the merger of jazz and rock created absolutely nothing of any long-term artistic value, I don't expect that a hybrid of jazz and rap will create anything of qualitative substance either."

Hip-hop certainly shares aspects of the jazz dance tradition: the themes, the emotion, the movement. The technique is different, pointed toes, high insteps, and ballet vocabulary are not as important to street dancers as to Broadway dancers. Some say hip-hop lacks "swing," rhythmic complexity, and the subtlety of classic jazz. The controversy of whether it is jazz or is not jazz dance will be settled only with the perspective of history.

Aerobic Dance

Aerobic dance is a phenomenon of the fitness boom that has brought the jazzy joy of moving to kinetic music to a wider population. Many nondancers have embraced the opportunity to move uninhibitedly in a safe, nurturing environment to exciting music. Recently, as more classes are being offered, participants have even had the opportunity to be selective in what kind of music they want to move to. Classes in Afro-Cuban aerobics, hip-hop aerobics, ballet aerobics, big band aerobics, oldies aerobics, and funk aerobics are appealing to individual jazz tastes.

Of course, the potential for injury is an enormous problem for beginning dancers who are finding some relatively inexperienced teachers pushing them too hard, too fast. One hopes that as the field matures, the wealth of scientific research and experience that traditionally trained dancers have accumulated over the past few years will help to curb the number of injuries common to aerobic dance. One hopes, too, that some of the information that is being gathered in aerobic dance research (such as the efficient and supportive design of the footwear) will spread to jazz dance classes.

Dance Synthesis: Ballet/Modern/Jazz

Just as European, African, and American arts merged to form jazz in the early part of this century and just as ballet, modern, and jazz dance techniques merged to form the professional jazz dancer of the second half of this century, the jazz dances of today are again influencing and being influenced by other forms of dance. This time, choreographers are taking the lead and reaching out for inspiration wherever they find it—from other dance styles and other countries. In 1991 in Chicago, the First World Jazz Dance Congress presented a concert that showcased international companies performing jazz dances heavily influenced by modern dance techniques and training. In 1992 in New York, Wynton Marsalis, artistic director of Jazz at Lincoln Center, collaborated with a modern choreographer (Garth Fagin) to create *Griot New York* and in 1993 with Peter Martins of the New York City Ballet to create a jazz ballet *en pointe: Jazz (Six Syncopated Movements)*. Though this is not only a recent phenomenon (Jerome Robbins is the undisputed master of jazz/ballet choreography since the fifties), the blending and overlapping of dance forms seems to be one identifiable trend that will continue into the next century.

Jazz Dance's Global Future

Molly Molloy, a London- and Paris-based American choreographer, offers the most inclusive definition of jazz dance:

> "Jazz dance is the twentieth-century version of everything that has gone before—every folk dance, every primeval expression of man. . . . I believe that jazz is anything that is happening today, and that includes crossing the street and turning the light up, turning your music on, and watching how life has a rhythm. Jazz dance is universal. It came from America—It's *American* jazz dance, known all over the world. But as I am a citizen of the world, as we all are, I see it more internationally. It is a reflection of popular culture, a popular culture that is worldwide."

Many jazz dance teachers claim that any new trend in jazz dance is unhealthy—that if it varies from historical definitions of jazz dance, it is a pollution of the jazz tradition. But, as we are seeing, the jazz-fog responds and shapes itself to cultural edifices and influences. Efforts to contain it, to limit it, to stop it are invariably frustrated by the collective, improvisatory, freedom-loving nature of the art. Jazz moves. It must move.

As to the other questions with which we began this chapter (Is jazz dance a serious art form? Is art, by definition, upper class or aristocratic? Is jazz dance really an American art form?) the authors will defer to two great jazz musicians. What they say about jazz music and jazz culture in general applies as well to jazz dance specifically:

> "The main argument against jazz has always been that it is not art. I think it is art, and a very special art. . . . Jazz goes on finding new paths, sometimes reviving old styles, but, in either case, looking for freshness. . . . Jazz is a fresh, vital art in the present tense, with a solid past and an exciting future."

Leonard Bernstein[9]

> "The city of jazz does not have any specific geographical location. It is anywhere and everywhere, wherever you can hear the sound, and it makes you do like this—you know! Europe, Asia, North and South America, the world digs this burg—Digsville, Gonesville, Swingersville, and Wailingstown. There are no city limits, no city ordinances, no policemen, no fire department . . .
>
> "In the city's public square, you find statues of heroes. They

appear to have been sculptured in bars, after-hours joints, and houses of ill-repute.

"I think I'll stay here in this scene, with these cats, because almost everybody seems to dig what they're talking about, or putting down. They communicate, Dad. Do you get the message?"

Duke Ellington[10]

Endnotes

1. Dizzy Gillespie with Al Fraser, *To Be, Or Not . . . to Bop*.
2. Though Siegenfeld was interviewed for this book, this particular quotation is taken from *Dance Teacher Now*, October 1990, 50.
3. Leonard Bernstein, *What Is Jazz* (CBS Records Omnibus Series). July 12, 1956.
4. Portia K. Maultsby, "West African Influences in U.S. Black Music," in *More than Dancing: Essays on Afro-American Music and Musicians*, ed. Irene V. Jackson.
5. The separation of body and mind in Western philosophy dates back to the Greeks but is most identified with Descartes. Today, some scientists and philosophers understand that the body and mind are one, but it's a difficult concept for some to accept. Dancers have understood this intuitively for a while. As Lynn Simonson says: "There is no separation between body and mind. I've been working toward this for many years. What I've been interested in—always—has been finding a way for the student to allow the whole person to emerge as a dancer."
6. Stanley Crouch, *Jazz Criticism and Its Effect on the Art Form*.
7. "The synthesis of European and African musical elements in the West Indies, the Caribbean, and in continental Latin America produced calypso, rumba, the tango, the conga, mambo, and so on, but not the blues and not ragtime, and not that extension, elaboration, and refinement of blues-break riffing and improvisation which came to be known as jazz." (Albert Murray, *Stomping The Blues*.)
8. Olly Wilson, "The Association of Movement and Music as a Manifestation of a Black Conceptual Approach to Music-Making," in *More than Dancing: Essays on Afro-American Music and Musicians*, ed. Irene V. Jackson.
9. Leonard Bernstein, *The Joy of Music*.
10. Duke Ellington, *Music Is My Mistress*.

CHAPTER 9

Jazz Dance Choreography

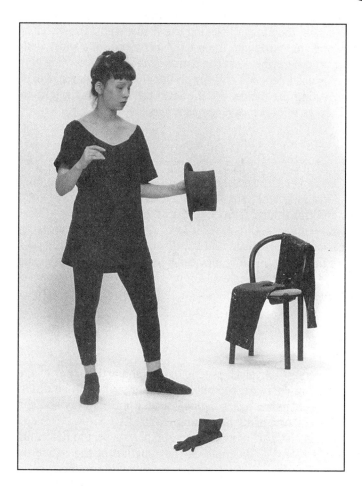

Outline

Choreography

Choreography is the art of composing dances. In its most restricted definition, choreography is the order of movements in a dance. In jazz choreography, these movements are often called *steps*.[1] When jazz dancers refer to learning the choreography of the dance, they mean learning the dance steps, the order of those steps, and how one step flows into the next (*transitions*). In a wider definition, "choreography" can describe what the dance is about and how it is performed. How the term is used depends entirely on the choreographer's level of responsibility when creating the dance. So, the term choreography might be defined, rather cyclically, as *what the choreographer does*.

Choreographer

The choreographer is the person who shapes the dance. He or she has final responsibility for determining what steps are done and in what order while inventing new steps and transitions as needed. Some choreographers—those who choreograph dance concerts, those well-known few who have achieved a certain level of success and/or respect, and some student choreographers—also control the entire dance production, including costuming, lighting, music arrangements, set design, and minute details of performance. The choreographer's degree of control is subject to the situation of the dance . . . subject to its *context*.

Context

Context is the dance's setting—physical, psychological, and artistic. For example, in each of the following contexts, the choreographer's role will be different—more or less comprehensive: a jazz dance concert; a Broadway show; a music video; a nightclub act; or a panty hose commercial.

The dance's function is also part of its context and plays a part in determining the choreographer's role. For example, is the function of the dance to: advance the story line of a play?; develop a character?; sell a product?; get a grade in choreography class?; or (with luck) be a work of art in itself?

Creative Team

Depending upon context, a choreographer may work alone or take part in a collaboration. In the commercial jazz dance world, the choreographer is very often part of a creative team assembled to realize a larger production—perhaps a stage show, a film, a revue, or a video. The creative team might include a costume designer, set designer, lighting designer, video editor, composer and/or music arranger, and writer.

The interaction among members of the team is fluid and changing. In dance concert work, the team is usually dedicated to helping the choreographer achieve his personal vision, but sometimes—especially in jazz dance—a choreographer is asked to create movement that serves another dominant vision. For example, a choreographer may be asked to provide steps and movement to animate a visual idea, as in Loie Fuller's early light shows, Paul Taylor's recent

Fuller *homage*, entitled *Oz*, or Walt Disney's *Mary Poppins* (choreography by Marc Breaux and Deedee Wood). The choreography may also be used:

- to demonstrate the beauty of a costume (e.g., some moments in Hanya Holm's *My Fair Lady* or a contemporary fashion show);
- to introduce the star of a revue (Tommy Tune's *Will Rogers Follies* or a Las Vegas revue);
- to move along the plot of a musical comedy (Agnes DeMille's *Oklahoma* or Susan Stroman's *Crazy for You*);
- to animate and sell a popular song (Paula Abdul's "Roll with It" or Michael Jackson and Michael Peters' "Thriller").

Choreographing

The term "choreographing" was first used to describe dance making in the commercial dance world by ballet master George Balanchine when he came to Broadway in 1936 with *On Your Toes*, the first of seventeen Broadway musicals he choreographed.[2] Until then, professional jazz choreographers on Broadway and in film were called, among other things, dance directors. They were often limited to supplying steps for the chorus line—a very different creative process from choreographing a unified whole dance idea. Featured dance stars such as Fred Astaire, Ray Bolger (the straw man in the *Wizard of Oz*), or the Nicholas Brothers did their own choreography.

When Balanchine started using the word, many directors and producers in the commercial theater and films resisted him, feeling the word was pretentious.[3] Nevertheless, the terms—choreographers, choreographing, choreography—took hold.

As "making up steps" evolved into choreographing, choreographers simultaneously gained more respect and responsibility within the creative team. Eventually, in the 1950s and 1960s, choreography dominated some shows, and some choreographers won the right to control the entire context of their dances. On Broadway, they became director-choreographers (Jerome Robbins, *West Side Story*; Michael Kidd, *Destry Rides Again*; and Michael Bennett, A *Chorus Line* and *Dream Girls*). Their works integrated dance, story, and characters and became known as *concept musicals*.

In the 1970s, 1980s, and 1990s, dance assumed a prominent place not only on Broadway (*Dream Girls, A Chorus Line, Dancin'; Jerome Robbins' Broadway, Jelly's Last Jam, Kiss of the Spider Woman,* and *Five Guys Named Moe, etc.*) but also in the merging music video medium and in dance films (*Flash Dance, Dirty Dancing, Strictly Ballroom,* and *Swing Kids*). Concert jazz dance gained audiences, too, though in America this context for jazz has not achieved its full potential commercially or artistically. Some exciting concert jazz dance companies include the Hubbard Street Dance Company and Danny Buraczeski Jazz Dance Company.

Jazz Choreography

Jazz choreography is identified as "jazz" by certain common elements it shares with jazz music.

- Jazz choreography is usually performed to jazz, rock, or pop music.
- Jazz choreography usually involves some sort of syncopation, rhythmic intricacy, or rhythmic play. Rhythm is emphasized by keeping the weight into the floor and through the use of body isolations.
- Jazz choreography usually includes some traditional jazz steps or jazz stylings.
- Jazz choreography usually centers upon various themes that are associated with jazz music and jazz culture. These themes might include frustration, physical and mental pain, fellowship, family, religion, poverty, love, sex, and drug and alcohol abuse. Jazz values often reflect a search for strength—either from God (as in gospels), from the beat (rap music, aerobics), from friends, family, stimulants, or from inner personal resources. Traditional jazz themes also include play and relaxation, call and response, and themes relevant to black America and black history: slavery, repression, life in the ghetto, freedom, anger, community, and religious faith. By far the most common theme in jazz dance is dance itself: movement play and movement playing with music.

Movement Shaped into Meaning

How does one choreograph a jazz dance?

1. Develop the *raw materials* of dance (steps, rhythms, transitions, stillness, music, and silence).
2. Master the *tools* of choreography (time, space, dynamics).
3. Using the choreographic tools, form and shape the raw material until it fits together and *means something*.

Sounds simple? It is . . . and it isn't. Anyone can follow steps one through three and come up with something that resembles a dance. But to come up with an actual dance—a work of art—each step must be enriched along the way as follows:

1. *Raw Materials:* To be artistically eloquent, the choreographer must have at his or her command a vast, internalized reserve of movement vocabulary and experience.
2. *Tools:* The choreographer should not just know about the choreographic tools of time, space, and dynamics, he or she must master them.
3. *Meaning:* The eventual meaning of the dance must be informed by a wisdom beyond the simplistic and must resonate in the minds and souls of the audience.

So that's it: With experience, skill, craft, courage, wisdom, and talent, a choreographer *shapes movement into meaning*.

Choreography: Movement Shaped Into Meaning.

1. MOVEMENT: Before one can write a story, one has to learn a language. Before one can make a dance, one has to have a basic movement vocabulary.
2. SHAPE: The raw materials of jazz dances are *shaped* into a syntax of movement and music. Shaping tools are: *time*, *space*, and *dynamics*.
3. MEANING: Meaning is what we are creating. It is achieved through the creative process, which includes the four stages of *Preparation*, *Incubation*, *Illumination*, and *Verification*.[4]

There's another complication along the winding path to choreography: choreography is not linear. At every point in the process, the choreographer must be open to surprises, be willing and eager to go back and start over, redo, followup, and throw out, and, always, be ruthless in exercising taste. This non-linear, seemingly unstructured creative process is perhaps most intimidating to aspiring choreographers. It may help for them to know that floundering—even failing—is a normal, expected, unavoidable part the process. The point is that choreography evolves and a good choreographer evolves with it, just as the choreographer herself evolves and good choreography evolves with her. Choreography is a system of expanding skills, so let's look at how those skills might be nurtured.

Developing Jazz Movement

For a jazz choreographer, fluency in jazz movement is as important as grammar and a vocabulary of words are for a writer. For writers, picking and choosing the appropriate word for the appropriate occasion is a sometimes conscious, sometimes unconscious, search into their past experiences with language: words, phrases, paragraphs, stories, literature, discourses, and English teachers. For dancers, choreography is a sometimes conscious, sometimes unconscious, search for the right movement based on all their past experiences with movement: dance classes, dance performances, films, television, videos, house parties, dance play in the studio, and dance teachers.

The dance class is an important resource for developing choreographic fluency. The *warm-up* trains the jazz dancer in traditional jazz "styles." The *vocabulary review* offers a wealth of traditional (vernacular) steps and variations. The combination part of the class is an apprenticeship for actual dance making: i.e., how steps fit or contrast to music, how new steps can be made from old, how one step evolves or breaks from the next, and how steps amplify or reflect rhythmic complexity. Stories, themes, and staging possibilities are also explored in class.

Movement vocabulary is also developed by watching as much dance as possible. Live performances are informative and inspiring—as much for the mistakes they illuminate as for the successes. Videotape is another valuable resource for the choreographer. Billy Siegenfeld, for one, studied videotapes of Fred Astaire, the Nicholas Brothers, and early Bob Fosse movies to develop his theater dance technique; and as we saw in the previous chapter, Susan Stroman credits her dance partner's exacting love of film musicals for much of her choreographic education.

Shaping with the Tools of Choreography

Though traditional jazz steps (see chapter 3) are used with pride as part of the tradition of jazz choreography, an important part of creating a dance is making it personal and unique. These personal touches identify an experienced choreographer. New steps and new variations on old steps are formed with the tools of choreography. As a painter uses oils, canvas, and brushes, a choreographer uses space, time, and dynamics.

Time

Perhaps the most important tool for jazz choreography, because of its intimate relationship to the music, is time. Time includes such elements as:

- *tempo* (how fast the music is played);
- *beat* (regular pulses underlying the music);
- *rhythm* (the recognizable pattern of the beats);
- *accent* (an emphasized beat);
- *meter* (the pattern of emphasized beats within a rhythm. [A duple meter will have a repeating pattern composed of one accented beat and one unaccented beat. A triple meter, or waltz time, will have one accented and two unaccented beats.]);
- *counts* (numbers that a choreographer assigns the beats, usually divided into sets of eight. These are a help in learning and remembering the dance pattern.);
- *syncopation* (rhythmic surprise [See Leonard Bernstein's eloquent description in chapter 8.]);
- *swing* (the polyrhythms that are unique to jazz and make the listener want to participate through movement).

If jazz is creative play, as many jazz masters describe it, then jazz timing may be approached as an intricate game. Aspects of rhythm and time might valuably be considered as *toys* to be played with in preparation for the final setting of the dance.

 Checklist: Time as a Tool

- A device to help find movement ideas.
- A device to adapt movement to dancers.
- A device for fitting the dance to its context.
- A device for fitting the dance to its music.
- A device for fitting the dance to its idea.
- As the subject of the dance itself.

Space

Space, as a choreographic tool, is a bit more complicated than one would think. It includes:

- *stage space or studio space* (the area in which the dance is set);
- *personal space* (the immediate space around the body)
- *interior space* (inside the dancer's body).

Space can be used as a tool to expand creative thinking about where movement takes place. For example, a beat can take place at the top of a leap as it travels halfway across the stage, or at the side of the body as a hip is thrown out to the side, or in the pit of the stomach where the audience can't see it, but where they will kinesthetically feel it, if it is sincerely performed. (For more on kinesthesia, see "performance" in chapter 10.)

 Checklist: Space as a Tool

While creating your dance, expand your thinking to include all space available to you. Not just big movements and small movements, but also:
- big movements in small spaces;
- small movements in big spaces;
- traveling (locomotor steps) through space;
- inner space (contractions or small pulses, even eyelash flickers);
- outer space;
- floor space;
- air space;
- wing space (the space just offstage);
- audience space.

Staging

The possibilities of space manipulation multiply when staging group works. The effect of even the slightest change of space will be magnified by the group. Space becomes "spaces," and the space *between* performers becomes charged with qualities of energy.

The power of individual space, so important in solo work, is reduced here. As an example, imagine a man standing in profile onstage. When he turns suddenly to face the audience, his presence, his energy is stronger. Now imagine twenty people all turning suddenly from profile to full-front. The effect is multiplied. In the "Material Girl"[5] music video, for example, twenty men in black tuxedos are standing in profile in a triangle around Madonna. In one sudden movement, they become twenty men in white shirts as they all turn front simultaneously. The viewer is stunned by the effect of so simple a movement when magnified by a masterful use of space, enhanced by costume.

Checklist: Groups in Space

Just by the grouping of people in space, powerful messages are sent to an audience.
- A group magnifies space when dancers move in unison.
- A group fractures space when dancers move separately.
- A group sends a societal message by its spacing:
    - One person moving in counterpoint is an individual;
    - Two people are a couple;
    - Three people hint that another group is forming.

Control of space is something that comes from experimentation and experience. A good place to start is with Doris Humphrey's classic book, *The Art of Making Dances*, written in 1959.[6] She categorized the areas of the stage according to their power. This chart is included here not as a definitive or limiting definition of stage-space psychology, but as a place to begin experiments in stage space.

"As a simple rule of thumb, there are six weak areas and seven strong ones on a stage (see diagram below). Also add the fact that movement, though personal on the footlights and therefore only suitable for intimate moods, loses power as it retreats upstage—except at dead center. Remember that the main paths which are illuminated, so to speak, are the diagonals and down the center; that the sides are very weak for either entrances or exits, or any movement. In fact, all places except the corners and center back are weak for emergences or departures. Innumerable studies can be devised to

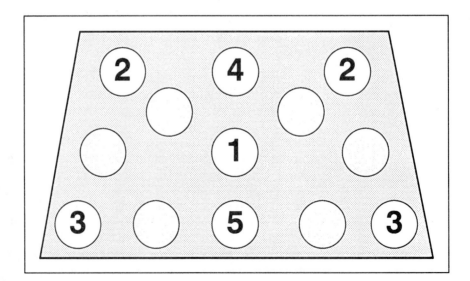

sample the flavor of these areas. Left far behind is the idea that a stage floor is just another kind of support, and it becomes more like a sensitive musical instrument to play on. I urge students not to think of it as static, but dynamic, full of vibration and sound, with the composer in control of the volume."

Dynamics

Though comprising elements of time and space, the dynamics tool is much more involved with energy. This includes the obvious: low energy and high energy, but also implicit are *qualities* of energy: gentle, sharp, angry, lyrical, contented, percussive, and fluid. Choreographers build dynamic values into their movement; and performers, too, must vary energy and style. Skilled phrasing of a dance combination is evidence of a dancer's fluency in dance dynamics. Brenda Bufalino says that phrasing is what made past dance greats like Honi Coles the acknowledged masters they were. She regrets that phrasing is not emphasized in classes today as much as it was in the past.

Choreographically, dances are usually more interesting when the dynamics are varied and include surprises and transitions. But, as usual in choreography this is not a "rule." Some very effective dances operate at one hypnotic energy level. The most famous example comes from ballet: In *La Bayadere*, one dancer after another steps out and does a slow *arabesque penché* until an entire company is onstage moving in perfectly shaped unison. It is a long, slow, breathtaking entrance with no dynamic change.

Classic jazz dance has its examples as well. In *Dancin'*, Bob Fosse choreographed a dance to "Big Noise from Winnetka" in which three jittery dancers twitched at one dynamic level for the entire piece.

A command of dynamics is, again, a matter of experience, confidence, and taste; however, there are some important hints for choreographers. The most important one follows:

> Don't rely too heavily on the music to determine your dance dynamic. It is very tempting to follow such a powerful guide, but jazz dance is described by some—including Luigi, Billy Siegenfeld, Brenda Bufalino, and many others—as rhythmic play with music, and playing *with* something implies a certain level of equality and challenge. Dance is a potent force in itself and shouldn't be sublimated to the music. Allow your dance some antagonism.

Dynamics can vary according to style and quality of movement as well as in the amount of energy used. Let's take simple anger as an example since, as Russell Clark points out, anger is the easiest emotion for beginning dancers or actors to simulate. Anger, in itself, is too vague a category to build a dance around. In exploring movement possibilities of anger, one can find a range of dynamic qualities if one is specific and open to different kinds of anger.

- defiance
- frustrated defiance
- victorious defiance
- pained anger
- sad anger

- enraged anger
- repressed anger
- hurt feelings and hurt bodies behind the anger
- protective anger
- defeated anger
- rage
- resentment
- annoyance
- depression
- pique

 Checklist: Using Dynamics as a Tool

Try:
- contrast;
- counterpoint;
- defiance;
- compliance
- force when the music is soft;
- quiet, or even stillness, when the music explodes;
- being an equal partner to the music;
- being its master;
- at times, being its slave.

Creating Meaning: The Creative Process

Now that we know where the vocabulary of jazz dance choreography comes from (movement experiences) and what tools are available for us to shape that vocabulary (space, time, dynamics), let's address the creative process itself: making meaning, making art.

In the past, creativity has seemed a rather mystical process attributable to the gods, to muses, to magic, or to miraculous inspiration. In this century, creativity has been subject to scientific research, and the results have thrown light into dark corners. While perhaps robbing art making of some of its mystery, science has made an important contribution to artists—particularly to young artists—by demystifying the experience. By intellectualizing creativity, researchers have made it less intimidating and more enabling, which is our primary purpose in presenting the following analysis.

Graham Wallace was the first to identify four stages in the creative process: Preparation, Incubation, Illumination, Verification. (In dance, we call this fourth stage "Polishing.") Let's examine how these stages relate to the art of choreography.

Preparation

According to Catherine Patrick, "Preparation is the time when the creative thinker is receiving or gathering his raw material."[7] The jazz choreographer's raw materials include primarily movement but may (depending on context) also include music preferences, personal ideas about costumes, lighting, stage context, set pieces, props, and other dancers.

Preparation is the most important step in the creative process. Studies on creativity in the arts have shown that the most successful artists (as determined by such criteria as originality, craftsmanship, and overall aesthetic value[8]) were those who spent the most time mulling over and exploring the raw materials of their potential product.

Researchers Getzels and Csikszentmihalyi labeled this kind of preparation "problem-formulating." They believe that in this "discovery-oriented behavior seemed to lie a key to the creative process."[9]

This "key to the creative process—this preparation phase—is also the most frustrating phase. The ability to swim comfortably in a sea of vague ideas, half-formed images, and movement possibilities is difficult, even frightening, to some people, but it is a decided asset to the choreographer.

(Because this phase of the choreographic process is so important, we have included as guide and example a series of Preparation Checklists as appendix H of this book.)

Incubation

Many famous thinkers and artists (Einstein, Poincaré, Picasso) have said their greatest insights have come after a period of long research (preparation), followed by a period of rest when they weren't thinking about their work at all. The change of state, from work to rest, seems to facilitate creativity.[10] There is much anecdotal evidence in creativity literature to suggest the desirability of allowing the subconscious mind to work with the raw materials of a problem for a while . . . after which comes "Illumination."

Illumination

Illumination is the "aha!" that comes after Incubation. A choreographer might find just the right theme, realize an eloquent ending or, as often happens, she may be seized by an unconscious force that seems to finish the dance almost in spite of herself. Make no mistake, this "miraculous" happening does not come from the muses nor does it come *without preparation*. Experienced choreographers will tell you that nine times out of ten, they struggle mightily with their dances and then that tenth dance will seemingly choreograph itself. It is usually a very good dance, too, but don't think that the effort expended on those nine other dances was "wasted." That tenth dance would not have been possible without the other nine struggles.

Verification

Verification, or polishing, refers to the meticulous work of making a creative idea presentable . . . tying up loose ends. This stage in the creative process might include reflecting on the totality of the dance to see if it's cohesive, if it fits together, if it "works." It may also include cleaning basic dance technique (rehearsing), finishing transitions, reworking any awkward areas of choreography, setting costumes, lights and stage sets, and finally placing the dance upon the dancers upon the stage. This part of the art is also part of the craft and is facilitated by a mastery of the choreographic tools: time, space, and dynamics. Polishing is not to be rushed. Details are important because it is confidence in each detail of a performing art that wins the trust of the audience. As the architect Mies van der Rohe put it, "God is in the details."

Endnotes

1. In ballet, steps are called *"pas"* and in modern dance, the term is resisted. Modern dance movement is organic movement that is developed and invented specific to each dance. Individual steps are not codified as part of a tradition-based lexicon; however, steps are taught in class as necessary "movement experience" and vocabulary building.
2. Richard Kislan, *Hoofing on Broadway: A History of Show Dancing* (New York: Prentice Hall Press, 1987).
3. Robert Alton illustrates this in an hilarious number in the film *White Christmas.* The dance was called "Choreography," and in it Danny Kaye satirized choreographic *artistes* in the context of a musical comedy.
4. Graham Wallace, *The Art of Thought*, 1926. Quoted in *The Creativity Question.* Albert Rothenberg and Carl R. Hausman (Durham, N.C.: Duke University Press, 1976).
5. The "Material Girl" video was choreographed by Ken Ortega after a famous production number choreographed for Marilyn Monroe by Jack Cole: "Diamonds Are a Girl's Best Friend" from *How to Marry a Millionaire.*
6. Doris Humphrey, *The Art of Making Dances*, (Pennington, N.J.: Princeton Book Co., 1987), 82.
7. Catherine Patrick, "Creative Thought in Artists," Journal Psychology (1937). The Journal Press, Provincetown, Mass. Quoted in *The Creativity Question*, ed.
8. The criteria of what is "creative" were established by Getzels and Csikszentmihalyi in a study of "successful" artists who were rated by a panel for "overall aesthetic value, originality, and craftsmanship." J. W. Getzels and M. Csikszentmihalyi, "The Creative Artist as an Explorer," Transaction Inc. from Human Intelligence, 1972 Transaction, Inc., 182–83, 187–92.
9. Ibid.
10. Rollo May, *The Courage to Create* (New York: Bantam Books, 1976).

CHAPTER 10

The Performance

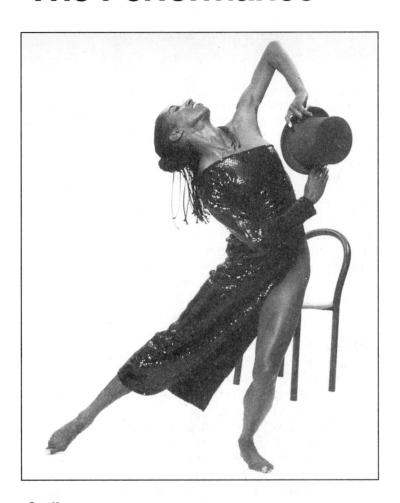

Outline

Jazz Dance: A Performing Art

Jazz dance is a performing art. Performance skills are an important part of jazz dance training.

> "Student performance in dance is not the dominant goal of the total dance curriculum, but it is part of the learning process of and about dance . . ."[1]

There are many reasons why performance skills are valuable to the jazz dancer. The Visual and Performing Arts Framework for California Public Schools, the highly regarded codification of dance pedagogical theory quoted above, includes the following:

> ". . . [Student performance in dance] is a significant culmination which encompasses creating, practicing, and working with others."

However valuable these experiences may be, many dancers may not have the opportunity to perform; some may feel intimidated by the thought of dancing for others or may feel that many years of training will be required before they are ready. Are performance techniques important to students who have no immediate intention of performing?

The answer is unequivocal: in jazz dance, techniques of performance should be an early and integral part of a jazz dancer's training, whether or not he or she ever plans to be on a stage. The reasons for this are embedded in the very definition of jazz dance.

The history and essence of jazz dance, as we've seen in chapter 8, reflect an integrating of body and mind and a sharing of artistic experience with others. The techniques of performance and communication (generally described here as presence, projection, and craft) are the very skills necessary to affirm such personal integration and communal sharing.

Performance skills are ways of understanding, enhancing, and communicating the dance. They are part of the discipline and artistic rigor that must be built into a dance and built into the dance artist from the first day of training.

Given the significance of such skills to the essential nature of jazz dance, it is unfortunate that so many dance students concentrate all of their class time on training the body as an "instrument"—an unnecessarily objectifying term—while virtually ignoring the psychological and social aspects of the art. Techniques of performance are not separate skills that are tacked on to the dance at the last minute before the dance is put upon the stage. Body, mind, and context should come together in jazz dance.

Teachers introduce performance techniques into their classes in a variety of ways, using a variety of words and descriptions. The vocabulary we will use in this chapter is a common, but not universal, one (e.g., "concentration" in lieu of "focus"). The introduction to this book provides an excellent example of one teacher's approach to integrating performance skills into technique training. In it, Luigi describes "feeling" as his primary goal in teaching jazz dance. He is not as concerned with the perfect *pirouette* as he is with enabling the student to *feel* the music, to *feel* the dancing, to *feel*, most importantly, what he, the dancer, is *feeling*.

"If a person has no feeling, it's because he has never looked inside himself; he has not found himself. It's there, but if he hasn't found it, then he's not a jazz dancer."

For Luigi, a jazz dancer is one who is in touch with his feelings, in other words, one who is centered—integrated—body and mind. It takes effort and discipline to look inside oneself. It takes effort and discipline to understand the dance. In class, it takes effort and discipline to focus on something beyond one's own two-dimensional mirror image. But one has to know what the goals of performance are. What does one focus on, on what does one expend effort, and to what standards does one maintain discipline?

In this chapter, we have taken Luigi's "feeling," Frank Hatchett's "VOP," Lynn Simonson's quest for "the emerging whole dancer," Billy Siegenfeld's "theater technique," along with other experts' descriptions of artistic goals, and analyzed the various steps and skills required to reach them. Though separated for purposes of discussion, the specific skills discussed here—concentration (focus), understanding, honesty, authority, and transcendence, as well as relaxation techniques, such as psychoneuromuscular training, visualization (see chapter 1), and preparation—typically work together to enhance and enrich the total dancer. In the process tension eases and stage fright becomes irrelevant. (An added benefit is that these performance and relaxation skills help in a more rapid and confident progress in the more physical aspects of dance technique as well.)

Through ....**relaxation** and preparation techniques,
one develops......................powers of **concentration,**
one enhances.....................**understanding,**
and encourages ....**honesty,**
and gains...........................**authority,**
which fosters ....**projection,**
and leads to ....**transcendence;**

which, in turn, leads to:

more controlled **relaxation,**
increased powers of **concentration,**
deeper **understanding,**
new level of **honesty,**
more confident **authority,**
more powerful **projection,**
a new **transcendence,**

and so on . . .

Presence

Before one can communicate through performance, one must learn to "be" onstage. The art of being onstage, openly and honestly, is called "presence." A stage is not a place one goes to hide. No amount of artifice or self-minimization will enable the person onstage to become invisible; therefore, a performer must learn to be comfortable onstage and comfortable revealing herself to other people.

How does one develop such ease? Conveniently, dancing helps. Dance releases inhibitions so that the more we dance, the less we fear and thus can reveal our inner self. The first tentative steps to such self-expression take place in the studio—in a safe and supportive jazz environment that is jazz's historical and natural context.

Another way of overcoming self-consciousness is to think, focus, and concentrate intently on something besides the self. The jazz dancer usually thinks about his music, and the more intricate the music, the easier it is to "lose oneself" in it—which is why many jazz dance teachers, among them Lynn Simonson, Billy Siegenfeld, Luigi, Danny Buraczeski, and Brenda Bufalino, emphasize the importance of using high-quality jazz compositions.

Projection

How does stage technique differ from classroom technique? Another way of asking that same question is: how does one move beyond display to communication? The answer is projection. It is achieved, as we've emphasized, through understanding, honesty, and concentration, which in turn leads to authority and transcendence, etc. We will look at each of these skills in turn, with the understanding that each aspect of performance enhances every other aspect. Dance artistry is, again, not a linear process.

Understanding the Dance

As we discussed in the last chapter, every dance is movement shaped into meaning. The meaning is not always a literal story line, but there is always a point of view and a structure (at least a beginning, a middle, and an end) that must be concretely understood by the performer. It is the theme or reason for the dance's existence. If the dancer does not understand her purpose onstage at every moment of the dance, she cannot convincingly speak to the audience.

Kinesthetic Intelligence   In addition to intellectual comprehension, a performer must also know the material *kinesthetically*. Kinesthetic intelligence[2] is the capacity we all have to know or understand something about ourselves and our world through internal, muscular, and physical senses and through movement. Understanding through movement is how someone in the audience responds directly and emotionally to a dance performance. On one level, that person sees, consciously understands, and reacts to the dance subject. But on a much more immediate and unconscious level, he or she feels what the dancer is feeling, body to body. In preparing for performance, then, the body must be given the time it needs to understand what it is doing without direction from the conscious mind. Achieving this "reflex" state of dance is necessary to the mastery of performance technique.

Variables of Performance   There are other aspects of dance that need to be rehearsed and internalized before a dance is performed: the effects of strong stage lights and shadows, costumes, makeup, spatial and personal relationships with other dancers, and the stage environment. These are the "variables of performance" that need to be integrated into the dance. Murray Louis, a modern choreographer of international acclaim, recently stated that "a dance doesn't become a dance until it's been performed many times. Opening night is simply a skeleton of the real dance."[3] He meant that the movements and the variables of performance in a dance must have time to blend into a delectable harmony that becomes subconscious with the rehearsal and performance experience. Only when it is subconscious will the audience react with their full complement of kinesthetic understanding and sympathy.

Elimination of the variables of performance and freedom from consciousness of physical surroundings also allow the dancer, while he is performing, to relinquish conscious control of the dance. This enables him to suspend the impediments of his internal critical judgment and the linear thought manipulations of an art form that is, in its essence, nonlinear and preconscious.

Honesty

An audience will not be fooled or manipulated. They can be surprised, they will be led, they can suspend belief for a time, but they resent being lied to or cheated. Therefore, a performer needs to build his performance on honesty, that is, his style must come from the material itself and not from superficial vanities or from old-fashioned show biz clichés. Trying to "sell" a dance, "turn on the charm," or "win over the audience" is a doomed road to mediocrity, and it is a road that is very hard to retrace.

Performance Clichés In 1977, Sammy Davis, Jr., one of the greatest jazz dancers ever, said that years of performing in nightclubs had led him to just such a dead end. Although still one of the great masters of his technique, he felt he had lost touch with his performance source, so for his Lincoln Center role in *Stop the World I Want to Get Off*, he set for himself the goal of finding motivation from the material, without relying on his repertoire of tried-and-true mannerisms. Many critics believed he was not successful in his goal, having realized his error too late in his performing career. The road back was too difficult. Gregory Hines, however, Davis's protégé, is not making the same mistake. He has fought hard to give his full attention to the dance itself, while resisting trite performance tricks. As he shows in his films *White Knights* and *Taps* and his Broadway show *Jelly's Last Jam*, a dance will *sell* itself if the performer is open and honest enough to allow it to shine through.

Mannerisms Another (very practical) reason for developing purity of form is that choreographers hire dancers who discipline their mannerisms. This was especially true of Bob Fosse. Although his choreography is very stylized and quirky, his auditions were simple and basic. He wanted pure technique and clean lines that he could control and manipulate to his own choreographic ends. Fosse was fond of Luigi-trained dancers,[4] and indeed his audition combination was very much in the controlled, clean, flowing Luigi style. (His audition combination can be seen in the opening sequence of the film *All That Jazz*.) Once the dancers were hired, he gave them Fosse-styled material (which was rather hunched, distorted, and isolated) with confidence that the dancers' mannerisms would not interfere with his own choreographic vision.

Concentration

Beginning performers often do not understand how the slightest deviation in internal concentration is communicated over vast theatrical distances and can significantly affect the audience's reaction to the dance. Onstage, a moment's lack of concentration on the dance or character, a moment's hesitation, self-consciousness, or insecurity is immediately sensed by the audience. The viewer's perception of such a lapse is often subconscious (kinesthetic); he is aware only of his sudden loss of confidence in the performer. If, for example, a dancer moves her arm through an arc in space, and halfway through the movement she stops thinking about the arc or the space (or whatever motivation there is for the movement) and starts thinking about her turnout, her abdominal muscles, or a too-strong sidelight, the audience will immediately sense the change in focus, even *if no measurable, physical change takes place in the dancer's body.* If the dance can't even keep the performer's attention, it will certainly lose the viewer's.

"Marking" Rehearsals   Full concentration in performance is so important and so difficult to achieve that it must be a part of every rehearsal, every workout, every class—even every mental rehearsal or visualization. Liza Minnelli, a consummate performer and excellent jazz dancer, is one professional who never "marks" or walks through a rehearsal, according to Susan Stroman, her choreographer:

> "Her work process is exceptional. She rehearses full-out. She sings full-out and dances full-out at all times. It's great for a choreographer. You can see your movement and know whether it is going to work right away. It's there onstage. She' a joy to work with."

As well as being a help to the choreographer, it is important to Minnelli's own performance. By the time the curtain goes up, she has fully integrated all the aspects of her performance.

Authority

Implicit in the audience member's presence in the theater is his desire to be somewhat changed: entertained, enlightened, relaxed, and/or emotionally moved. The performer must take responsibility for this change. If the dancer understands his material, has developed the concentration to focus on its importance, and has honestly put his trust in the dance, then he is ready to put forth his case with authority. The good performer leads, and the audience must have confidence in his leadership to be moved.

Transcendence

There is one more point that must be emphasized: during a performance, the dancer must not think about any of this. Magical performances occur when a performer is free from censorship, that is, not instructing herself or judging herself as she's dancing. Ideally, she should not even be *aware* of herself. The performance skills that have been discussed here—understanding, honesty, concentration, authority—can become subconscious, just as movements can be if they are practiced enough. When the dancer has achieved control over these psychological and physical skills, what is she thinking about then? Nothing. She has reached the transcendent state that Luigi refers to: she is feeling.

Performance Craft

When a dancer has confidence in his dance technique, confidence in the steps given by the choreographer, confidence in his own personality (enough to be able to reveal all of it), confidence in his power to move the audience—and has learned to project his confidence—he is well on the path to mastery of dance performance. There are other devices of performance technique that help the mind and body integrate to perform, certain techniques that are part of the performer's craft.

Preparation

The moments just before entering onstage should be a time of internal preparation. There are many devices a dancer can use to prepare for a performance, such as relaxation techniques, mental rehearsal, and visualization. Some dancers use the ritual of the warm-up as a time for solitary contemplation of the psychological as well as physical demands of the upcoming performance. Some professional dancers, believe it or not, refuse to talk for several hours before a performance so that they can become fully centered in the nonverbal centers of their brains. Some jog so that the regular rhythms of their body will balance the tension between body and mind. Experience will determine what methods work best for you.

Body Image

Of course, the performing dancer wants a perfectly tuned and responsive body, and that is one of the major goals of dance training, but it must be emphasized that entirely too much emphasis has been put on an imaginary "ideal dancer's shape." An "ideal" body is a myth, a destructive myth, that has destroyed many careers and lives.

Gelsey Kirkland reports in her biography, *Dancing on My Grave*, that she wasted a lot of her career, perhaps never achieving her full potential because of time, money, and emotional strength wasted on trying to look like, act like, and dance like Suzanne Farrell, whom she considered to be the "ideal" ballerina. She had useless, destructive plastic surgery and eventually turned to drugs because, among other things, she was not able to transform herself into someone else. The tragedy is that she lost years of being Gelsey Kirkland, who many critics believe was the greatest ballerina of the time. Placing too much credence in such an ideal ultimately undermines confidence in the instrument one has to work with, which is certain to be the best instrument for conveying the performer's personal artistic motivation.

Another example: In the 1960s, Rudolf Nureyev was hailed as the greatest male ballet dancer of his time.[5] He was tall, elegant, stately and long-limbed—the perfect Prince Charming. A few years later, Mikhail Baryshnikov replaced him as the "greatest"—short, boyish, short-legged. Baryshnikov was

Nureyev's opposite in every way and still achieved the pinnacle of success in his field.

It is true that some choreographers—usually choreographers who tend to see dancers as instruments rather than artists—prefer using certain body types to reflect their choreography. George Balanchine and Alwin Nikolais prefer thin, long-limbed dancers, but Twyla Tharp looks more at personalities, and Maurice Bejart considers sex appeal. What's important to learn is that different choreographer's tastes are their own personal biases and do not reflect concrete universal aesthetic standards. In fact, Luigi believes that today's choreographers are making a mistake in emphasizing choreography over the individual dancer.

> "Choreographers in the past, like Robert Alton, Jerome Robbins, and Gene Kelly, used choreography to make the dancer look good. Today's choreographers use dancers to make the choreography look good. The result is a decline in the art of jazz dance as a personal statement, which is reflected in the fact that there are very few well-known dancers today as compared with the past."

The jazz dancer's priority is to develop his own, unique artistry and to use his instrument to its full potential—with confidence.

Coping with Stage Fright

Experience is the best—the only—way to fully control stage fright. There is an ancient show biz belief that all performers should feel some nervousness before a performance in order to give their performance "an edge." That might be true for veteran performers who feel a more practiced, personally familiar form of stage fright. But, for theatrical novices who are dealing, in many cases, with outright panic, this is not as valid a point. Nervousness onstage for a dancer can be very destructive. It saps confidence, distracts concentration, and makes muscles quiver—which during a one-legged balance is not a pretty sight. As we have said before, any personal reaction, emotion, or feeling onstage not relevant to the subject of the dance is a distraction the audience will sense. Therefore stage fright must be confronted and channeled.

Techniques for handling stage fright are *precisely the same techniques* described in this chapter for enhancing performance and described in the first chapter for preparing for the jazz dance class: relaxation and visualization techniques reduce stress; and confidence is enhanced through understanding, honesty, concentration, authority, transcendence, preparation, self-knowledge, and . . . more confidence.

Checklist: Performing with Confidence

- *Understanding:* Understand exactly what you are doing onstage. Understanding the dance will relieve the doubts you may have of your performance mission.
- *Honesty:* Deal with the dance directly and honesty. Avoid the temptation to depend on the illusion of tacked-on charm or phony smiles. One cannot have confidence in an illusion.
- *Concentration:* Develop your powers of concentration during class and during rehearsals so that you can focus on the dance instead of the fear.
- *Authority:* Understand your responsibility to take control of the event. If you are the master of the moment, you will not be concerned during the actual dance with how the audience is judging you.
- *Confidence:* Build your confidence by eliminating all possible physical variables during rehearsal. Know your stage, your dance, your makeup, your costumes, and your lighting in advance so that you can free your mind to enjoy the performance experience.
- *Preparation:* Make time for the full ritual of entering into the dream. Be a prepared and relaxed dancer before you enter the actual dance.

Endnotes

1. California State Department of Education, Visual and Performing Arts Framework and Criteria Committee, *Visual and Performing Arts Framework for California Public Schools: K through Grade 12*, Janet Lundin and Theodore Smith, eds., 1982.
2. Howard Gardner, *Frames of Mind: The Theory of Multiple Intelligences* (New York: Basic Books, 1985).
3. Murray Louis, phone interview, New York, March 20, 1991.
4. "I have known and respected Luigi for quite some time as one of the most capable and talented dance teachers in New York. His standards have always been held in the highest esteem by all in the dance world." (Bob Fosse, personal correspondence, 7/10/87)
5. Clive Barnes, "A Man Named Rudolph," *Dance Magazine*, May 1990.

Basic Musculature Chart

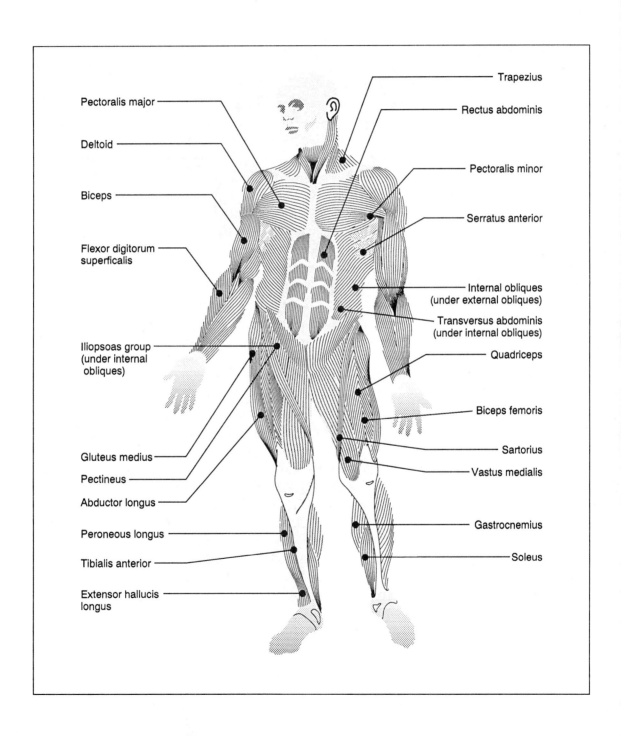

Trapezius

Pectoralis major

Rectus abdominis

Deltoid

Pectoralis minor

Biceps

Serratus anterior

Flexor digitorum superficalis

Internal obliques (under external obliques)

Transversus abdominis (under internal obliques)

Iliopsoas group (under internal obliques)

Quadriceps

Biceps femoris

Gluteus medius

Sartorius

Pectineus

Vastus medialis

Abductor longus

Peroneous longus

Gastrocnemius

Tibialis anterior

Soleus

Extensor hallucis longus

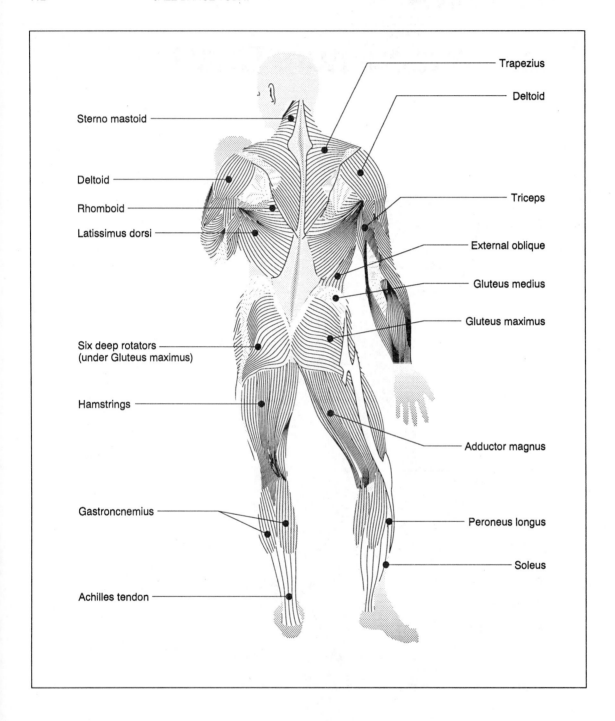

Trapezius

Deltoid

Sterno mastoid

Triceps

Deltoid

Rhomboid

Latissimus dorsi

External oblique

Gluteus medius

Gluteus maximus

Six deep rotators
(under Gluteus maximus)

Hamstrings

Adductor magnus

Gastroncnemius

Peroneus longus

Soleus

Achilles tendon

Essential Information on Vitamins and Minerals

Name	Solubility	RDA	Functions	Deficiencies and excesses	Sources
A	Fat soluble Stored in body	5,000 units (men) 4,000 units (women) Toxic level: 25,000 to 50,000 units daily	1. Formation of body tissue 2. Development of mucous secretions in nose, mouth, digestive tract, organs (which) show bacterial entry) 3. Development of visual purple in the retina of the eye—which allow one to see in the dark 4. Produces the enamel producing cells of the teeth 5. Assists normal growth	Deficiencies can cause night blindness, damaged intestinal tract, damaged reproductive tract, scaly skin, poor bones, dry mucous membranes, and in children, poor enamel in the teeth Toxic symptoms (of Retinol): may mimic brain tumor (increased pressure inside the skull), weight loss, irritability, loss of appetite, severe headaches, vomiting, itching, menstrual irregularities, diarrhea, fatigue, skin lesions, bone and joint pains, loss of hair, liver and spleen enlargement, and insomnia. In children, overdose can stunt growth	Carrots Yellow fruits Green leafy vegetables Butter and margarine Whole milk Liver Fish Fortified nonfat milk Ripe tomatoes Egg yolks
B–1 (thiamin)	Water soluble	1.5 mg (men) 1.2 mg (women)	1. Metabolizes carbohydrates 2. Resulting glucose (sugar) nourishes muscles and nerves	Deficiencies can cause: mental depression, moodiness, quarrelsomeness and uncooperativeness, fatigue, irritability, lack of appetite, muscle cramps, constipation, nerve pains (due to degeneration of myelin sheath which covers the nerves), weakness and feeling of heaviness in the legs, beri-beri (a disease in which the muscles atrophy and become (paralyzed)	Liver Pork Yeast Organ meats Whole grains Bread Wheat germ Peanuts Milk Eggs Soy beans

Name	Solubility	RDA	Functions	Deficiencies and excesses	Sources
B–2 (riboflavin)	Water soluble	1.8 mg (men) 1.4 mg (women)	Effects rate of growth and metabolic rate since it is necessary for the cell's use of protein, fat, and carbohydrate	Deficiencies can cause: burning and itching eyes, blurred and dim vision, eyes sensitive to light, inflammation of the lips and tongue, lesions at the edges of the mouth, digestive disturbances, greasy, scaly skin	Eggs Liver and other organs Yeast Milk Whole grains Bread Wheat germ Green leafy vegetables
B–3 (niacin or nicotinic acid)	Water soluble Limited storage in body	18 mg (men) 14 mg (women)	1. Similar to riboflavin in metabolizing foods (especially sugars) 2. Maintains normal skin conditions 3. Aids in functioning of the gastrointestinal tract	Deficiencies can cause: Dermatitis (red, tender skin, becoming scaly and ulcerated), fatigue, sore mouth (tongue), diarrhea, vomiting, nervous disturbances, mental depression, anorexia, weight loss, headache, backache, mental confusion, irritability, hallucinations, delusions of persecution, pellagra. Large doses can be toxic because it dilates blood vessels. Can cause skin flushing, dizziness, head throbbing, also—dryness of skin, itching, brown skin pigmentation, decreased glucose (sugar) tolerance and perhaps a rise in uric acid in the blood	Yeast Liver Wheat bran Peanuts Beans
Pantothenic acid	Water soluble Little storage in body	10 mg	1. Carbohydrate, fat and protein metabolism 2. Synthesis of cholesterol and steroid hormones 3. Aids the functioning of the adrenal cortex 4. Aids in choline metabolism	Almost never deficient in human diets. Various animal studies have shown different results from deficiency: rough skin, diarrhea, anemia, possible coma convulsions, hair loss, and many other symptoms. But they have not been shown in humans	Liver Organ meats Eggs Yeast Wheat bran Legumes Cereals
Biotin	Water soluble	No RDA	Metabolism of amino acids, fatty acids and carbohydrate	Deficiencies are extremely rare. Raw egg whites (which combine with the biotin in the intestines and make it unavailable and some antibiotics (which kill the	Manufactured in the intestines Also found in: liver yeast kidney egg yolks

Name	Solubility	RDA	Functions	Deficiencies and excesses	Sources
				biotin producing organisms in the intestines) could cause a deficiency	
				Deficiency would be marked by: dry, scaly skin, gray pallor (skin color) slight anemia, muscular pains, weakness, depression and loss of appetite	
B–6 (pyridoxine)	Water soluble	2.0 mg (men) 2.0 mg (women)	1. Catalyst in protein, fat, and carbohydrate metabolism. A high protein diet increases the need for B–6 2. Converts tryptophan to niacin 3. Assists in nervous system	Anemia, dizziness, nausea, vomiting, irritability, confusion, kidney stones, skin and mucous membrane problems. In infants: irritability, muscle twitching, convulsion. Excesses—impaired sensation in limbs. Unsteady gait.	Usually not necessary to supplement Wheat germ Kidney Liver Ham Organ meats Legumes Peanuts
Folic acid (folacin)		400 mcgm	1. Aids in maturation of red and white blood cells 2. May assist in the synthesis of nucleic acids	Blood disorders, anemia, diarrhea Deficiencies most likely to occur during pregnancy and lactation	Yeast Liver Egg yolk Green leafy vegetables
B–12	Water soluble Stored in the body	6.0 mcgm (men & women)	1. Controls blood forming defects and nerve involvement in pernicious anemia 2. Involved in protein, fat, carbohydrate, nucleic acid and folic acid metabolism 3. Necessary to the normal functioning of cells, especially in the bone marrow, nervous system and intestinal tract	Sore tongue, amenorrhea, signs of degeneration of the spinal cord, anemia, heart and stomach trouble, headache, and fatigue	Liver Organ meats Oysters Salmon Eggs Beef Milk

Name	Solubility	RDA	Functions	Deficiencies and excesses	Sources
C (ascorbic acid)	Water soluble Little body storage	45 mg (men) 45 mg (women) 10 mg per day prevents scurvy	1. Forms collagen intracellular cement which strengthens cell walls (especially the small blood vessels and capillaries), tooth dentine, cartilage, bones, and connective tissue 2. Aids in the absorption of iron 3. Aids in formation of red blood cells in the bone marrow 4. Aids in the metabolism of some amino acids (phenylalanine and tyrosine) 5. May be involved in the synthesis of steroid hormones from cholesterol 6. Any body stress may deplete the vitamin C in the tissues—shock, fracture, or bacterial infections	Scurvy results from low vitamin C intake. Minor symptoms of vitamin C deficiency could be: subcutaneous hemorrhages (bleeding below the skin), bleeding from gums, swollen gums Excess of Vitamin C can result in kidney stones and diarrhea, destruction of B–12, acidoses	Citrus Fresh fruits Berries Broccoli Tomatoes Green leafy vegetables Baked potatoes Turnips
D	Stored in liver Fat soluble	400 units Toxic level 1,000 to 1,500 units	1. Assists in the development of bones and teeth by aiding calcium to harden 2. Facilitates the absorption of calcium and phosphorus, lack of which can cause muscular cramping	Deficiencies: ricketts (children), osteomalacia (women who have had frequent pregnancies and poor diets). Teeth may be more susceptible to caries (cavities). Cramping in muscles if there is a low level of calcium or phosphorus in the blood. Soft bones, bowed legs, poor posture Toxic symptoms: fatigue, weight loss, nausea, vomiting, weakness,	Exposure to ultraviolet light (sunlight) can give minimum daily requirements by changing one type of cholesterol to vitamin D Milk Fish liver oils Egg yolk Butter Whole milk

Name	Solubility	RDA	Functions	Deficiencies and excesses	Sources
				headache, kidney damage, kidney stones, hardening of the soft tissues of the heart, blood vessels, lungs, stomach and kidneys. Increases cholesterol level of blood. Makes bone more fragile. High levels in developing fetuses and young children may cause mental retardation or blood vessel malformation (especially a blockage in the aorta—the major artery from the heart)	Nonfat milk (with D) Margarines (with D added)
E	Fat Soluble not stored in body	15 units	Unknown. It is thought to stabilize membranes. May be helpful in stabilizing Vitamin A. May be necessary in diets high in polyunsaturated fats	No known deficiency symptoms in human adults. Some premature infants apparently do not immediately develop the ability to absorb the vitamin	Synthesized in the intestines. Alpha tocopherol E probably better than mixed-tocopherol E. Human milk (cow's milk poor) Margarine Oil salad dressing Vegetable oils Nuts Eggs Cereal germ Green leafy vegetables
K	Fat soluble	Probably 30–50 mcgm	Helps in the production of prothrombin (blood clotting agent)	Antibiotics taken orally (which could kill the synthesizing bacteria) or diarrhea (which could flush out the bacteria) could possibly cause a deficiency Newborn infants, especially premature babies, often suffer from a deficiency. This may cause excessive bleeding Toxic symptoms in infants: jaundice, mild anemia	Synthesized by intestinal bacteria Green leafy vegetables Cabbage Liver Cauliflower Smaller amounts in: tomatoes, egg yolk and whole milk

Name	Solubility	RDA	Functions	Deficiencies and excesses	Sources
Calcium		800 mg (men & women)	Development of strong bones and teeth. Help muscles contract and relax normally. Utilization of iron. Normal blood clotting. Maintenance of body neutrality. Normal action of heart muscle	Rickets, porous bones, bowed legs, stunted growth, slow clotting of blood, poor tooth formation, tetany	Milk, cheese, mustard, turnip greens, clams, oysters, broccoli, cauliflower, cabbage, molasses, nuts. Small amount in egg, carrot, celery, orange, grapefruit, figs, and bread made with milk
Fluorine		One part per million in water Toxic at 6 to 10 ppm	Resistance to dental caries Deposition of bone calcium May be involved in iron absorption	Deficiencies: weak teeth and bones, anemia, impaired growth. At levels of 1.5 to 4 parts per million teeth will be strong, but may be mottled. At levels over 6 ppm teeth and bones may be deformed	Water supply containing 1 ppm. Small amount in many foods
Iodine		0.1 mg (men & women)	Constituent of thyroxine which is a regulator of metabolism	Enlarged thyroid gland Low metabolic rate Stunted growth Retarded mental growth	Iodized salt Sea foods Foods grown in nongoiterous regions
Iron		10 mg (men) 18 mg (women)	Constituent of hemoglobin, which carries oxygen to the tissues	Nutritional anemia, pallor, weight loss, fatigue, weakness, retarded growth	Red meats, especially liver, green, vegetables, yellow fruits, prunes, raisins, legumes, whole grain and enriched cereals, molasses, egg yolk, potatoes, oysters.
Magnesium		350 mg (men) 300 mg (women)	Activates various enzymes. Assists in breakdown of phosphates and glucose necessary for muscle constractions. Regulates body temperature. Assists in synthesizing protein	Failure to grow, pallor weakness, irritability of nerves and muscles, irregular heartbeat, heart and kidney damage, convulsions and seizures, delirium, depressions	Soya flour, whole wheat, oatmeal, peas, brown rice, whole corn, beans, nuts

Name	Solubility	RDA	Functions	Deficiencies and excesses	Sources
Phosphorus		800 mg (men & women)	Development of bones and teeth. Multiplication of cells. Activation of some enzymes and vitamins. Maintenance of body neutrality. Participates in carbohydrate metabolism	Rickets, porous bones, bowed legs, stunted growth, poor tooth formation. Excesses of phosphorus may have same effect on the bones as deficient calcium (osteoporosis—porous bones)	Milk, cheese, meat, egg yolk, fish, nuts, whole grain cereals, legumes, soya flour, whole wheat, oatmeal, peas, brown rice, whole corn, beans
Potassium		2.5 grams	Acid-base balance. Carbohydrate metabolism. Conduction of nerve impulses Contraction of muscle fibers. May assist in lowering blood pressure (if consumed in equal proportions as sodium)	Apathy, muscular weakness, poor gastrointestinal tone, respiratory muscle failure, tachycardia (irregular heartbeat), cardiac arrest (heart stops beating)	Soybeans, cantaloupe, sweet potato, avocado, raisins, banana, halibut, sole, baked beans, molasses, ham, mushrooms, beef, white potatoes, tomato, kale, radishes, prune juice, nuts and seeds, wheat germ, green leafy vegetables, cocoa, vegetable juices, cream of tartar, prunes, figs, apricots, oranges, grapefruit
Sodium		1–2 grams (1/5 to 2/5 teaspoon)	Constituent of extracellular fluid. Maintenance of body neutrality. Osmotic pressure. Muscle and nerve irritability	Muscle cramps, weakness, headache, nausea, anorexia, vascular collapse Excess may raise blood pressure	Sodium chloride (table salt) Sodium bicarbonate (baking soda) Monosodium glutamate (Accent) The greatest portion of sodium is provided by table salt and salt used in cooking. Foods high in sodium

Name	Solubility	RDA	Functions	Deficiencies and excesses	Sources
					include: dried beef, ham, canned corned beef, bacon, wheat breads, salted crackers, flaked breakfast cereals, olives, cheese, butter, margarine, sausage, dried fish, canned vegetables, shellfish and salt water fish, raw celery, egg white.
Zinc		15 mg	Metabolism, formation of nucleic acid	Impaired growth, sexual development, skin problems	Beef, chicken, fish, beans

Calorie/Activity Chart

Caloric Output for Exercising

ACTIVITY	*CALORIES/MINUTE	ACTIVITY	*CALORIES/MINUTE
BADMINTON	5.0- 7.5	GYMNASTICS	5.0
BASEBALL	2.4- 4.0	balancing	2.5
BASKETBALL	8.6	abdominal	3.0
BOWLING	4.0- 5.0	trunk bending	3.5
CANOE ROWING		hopping	6.5
slow (2-3mph)	2.0- 3.0	HANDBALL	10.0-13.3
moderate (4mph)	5.0- 7.0	HOCKEY	12.0-15.0
rapid (5-6 mph)	7.0- 8.0	HORSEBACK RIDING	3.0- 9.5
CLASSWORK (reading)	1.0- 2.0	JOGGING (slow)	10.0-15.0
CLIMBING	10.7- 13.2	RECLINING	1.5- 1.6
CYCLING		ROPE SKIPPING	12.0
5 mph	4.5	RUNNING	
9 mph	7.0	7 mph	10.0
13 mph	11.1	9 mph	11.0
DANCING (continuous—*not* class)		12 mph	14.5-19.4
slow	3.0	SHIVERING	5.0- 7.0
fast	4.0- 7.0	SKATING	
DOMESTIC WORK		ice	6.6
bed making	3.5	roller	7.8-13.0
dusting	2.5	SKIING (CROSS COUNTRY)	
ironing	1.7	moderate speed	10.0-16.0
meal preparation	2.5	maximum speed	15.0-19.0
cleaning floors	3.5	SLEEPING	1.0- 1.2
standing	2.6	SQUASH	10.0-11.0
typing	1.6	SWIMMING	
washing	2.6	breaststroke	11.0
DRESSING	1.5- 2.0	backstroke	11.5
DRIVING A CAR	2.0	crawl	14.0
EATING	2.0	TALKING	1.0- 1.2
FARM CHORES	2.0- 3.0	TENNIS	7.1- 7.5
FENCING	5.0	table	5.0
FOOTBALL		WALKING	
touch	8.9	2 mph	2.5
tackle	12.0	3 mph	3.5
GOLF	5.0	5 mph	5.5
		up stairs	10.0-12.0
		WRESTLING	7.0- 9.0

*3500 Calories equals 1 pound

Energy Equivalents

Minutes of participation in the activities listed at right needed to expend the calorie energy of the foods listed below.	Calorie content	Reclining	Walking	Bicycle Riding	Swimming	Running
Beverages						
Carbonated, 8 oz. glass	106	82	20	13	9	5
Ice cream soda, chocolate	255	196	49	31	23	13
Malted milkshake, chocolate	502	386	97	61	45	26
Milk, 8 oz. glass	166	128	32	20	15	9
Milk, skim, 8. oz. glass	81	62	16	10	7	4
Milkshake, chocolate	421	324	81	51	38	22
Beer, 8 oz. glass	114	88	22	14	10	6
Wine, 3 1/2 oz. glass	84	65	16	10	8	4
Desserts						
Cake, 2 layer	356	274	68	43	32	18
Cookie, chocolate chip	51	39	10	6	5	3
Doughnut	151	116	29	18	13	8
Ice cream, 1/6 Qt.	193	148	37	24	17	10
Gelatin, with cream	117	90	23	14	10	6
Pie, apple, 1/6	377	290	73	46	34	19
Sherbet, 1/6 Qt.	177	136	34	22	16	9
Strawberry shortcake	400	308	77	49	36	21
Fruit & Fruit Juices						
Apple, large	101	78	19	12	9	5
Banana, small	88	68	17	11	8	4
Orange, medium	68	52	13	8	6	4
Peach, medium	46	35	9	6	4	2
Apple juice, 8 oz. glass	118	91	23	14	10	6
Orange juice, 8 oz. glass	120	92	23	15	11	6
Tomato juice, 8 oz. glass	48	37	9	6	4	2
Meats						
Bacon, 2 strips	96	74	18	12	9	5
Ham, 2 slices	167	128	32	20	15	9
Pork chop, loin	314	242	60	38	28	16
Steak, T-bone	235	184	45	29	21	12

Minutes of participation in the activities listed at right needed to expend the calorie energy of the foods listed below.	Calorie content	Reclining	Walking	Bicycle Riding	Swimming	Running
Miscellaneous						
Bread & butter, 1 slice	78	60	15	10	7	4
Cereal, dry 1/2 c. w/milk, sugar	200	154	38	24	18	10
French dressing, 1 tbsp.	59	45	11	7	5	3
Mayonnaise, 1 tbsp.	92	71	18	11	8	5
Pancake, with syrup	124	95	24	15	11	6
Spaghetti, 1 serving	396	305	76	48	35	20
Cottage cheese, 1 tbsp.	27	21	5	3	2	1
Poultry & Eggs						
Chicken, fried 1/2 breast	232	178	45	28	21	12
Chicken "TV dinner"	542	217	104	66	48	28
Turkey, 1 slice	130	100	25	16	12	7
Egg, fried	110	85	21	13	10	6
Egg, boiled	77	59	15	9	7	4
Sandwiches & Snacks						
Club	590	454	113	72	53	30
Hamburger	350	269	67	43	31	18
Roast beef with gravy	430	331	83	52	38	22
Tunafish salad	278	214	53	34	25	14
Pizza, with cheese, 1/8	180	138	35	22	16	9
Potato chips, 1 serving	108	83	21	13	10	6
Cheddar cheese, 1 oz.	111	85	21	14	10	6
Seafood						
Clams, 6 medium	100	77	19	12	9	5
Cod, steamed, 1 piece	80	62	15	10	7	4
Crabmeat, 1/2 cup	68	52	13	8	6	4
Haddock, 1 piece	71	55	14	9	6	4
Halibut steak, 1/4 lb.	205	158	39	25	18	11
Lobster, 1 medium	50	38	10	6	4	3
Shrimp, french fried, 1 serv.	180	138	35	22	16	9
Vegetables						
Beans, green, 1 cup	27	21	5	3	2	1
Beans, canned, 1/2 cup	38	29	7	5	3	2
Carrot, raw	42	32	8	5	4	2
Lettuce, 3 large leaves	30	23	6	4	3	2
Peas, green, 1/2 cup	56	43	11	7	5	3
Potato, boiled, 1 medium	100	77	19	12	9	5
Spinach, fresh, 1/2 cup	20	15	4	2	2	1

SUGGESTED WEIGHT

HEIGHT[1]	WEIGHT IN POUNDS[2]	
	19 to 34 years	35 years and over
5'0"	97-128[3]	108-138
5'1"	101-132	111-143
5'2"	104-137	115-148
5'3"	107-141	119-152
5'4"	111-146	122-157
5'5"	114-150	126-162
5'6"	118-155	130-167
5'7"	121-160	134-172
5'8"	125-164	138-178
5'9"	129-169	142-183
5'10"	132-174	146-188
5'11"	136-179	151-194
6'0"	140-184	155-199
6'1"	144-189	159-205
6'2"	148-195	164-210
6'3"	152-200	168-216
6'4"	156-205	173-222
6'5"	160-211	177-228
6'6"	164-215	182-234

[1] Without shoes.

[2] Without clothes.

[3] The higher weights in the ranges generally apply to men, who tend to have more muscle and bone; the lower weights more often apply to women, who have less muscle and bone.

Adapted from
"Nutrition and Your Health: Dietary Guidelines for Americans," 3rd ed., 1990, U.S. Department of Agriculture, U.S. Department of Health and Human Services.

Dance Publications and Journals

Attitude: The Dancer's Magazine
1040 Park Place
Brooklyn, NY 11213-1946

**American Alliance for Health,
Physical Education, Recreation
and Dance (AAHPERD)
Publications Catalog** *and* **JOPERD**
(The Journal of Physical Education,
Recreation and Dance)
1900 Association Drive
Reston, VA 22091
703-476-3400

**American Council for the
Arts Catalog**
(Publishers and distributors of trade
and professional books in the arts
for 25 years.)
c/o ACA Books
American Council for the Arts
Department 32
1 East 53rd Street
New York, NY 10022

CORD/Dance Research Journal
(Congress of Research for Dance)
New York University Dance Dept.,
Education 684D
35 West 4th Street, Room 675
New York, NY 10003
212-998-5400

Dance Book Club
12 West Delaware Avenue
Pennington, NJ 08534
800-326-7149

Dance Directory
Information on dance major and
minor programs across the country.
Available through the AAHPERD
(Address above)

Dance Ink
145 Central Park West
New York, NY 10133-0212
212-826-9607

Dance Magazine, Inc.
33 West 60th Street
New York, NY 10023
212-245-9050

The Dance Mart
(Rare books, magazines, autograph
material, and other collectibles per-
taining to dance.)
Box 48, Homecrest Station
Brooklyn, NY 11229

Dance Pages
P.O. Box 916, Ansonia Station
New York, NY 10023-0916
212-869-2101

Dance Resource Guide
A compilation of resources for dance,
including music, recording compa-
nies, books, journals, multicultural
resources, dance organization, and
more!
Available through the American
Alliance for Health, Physical
Education, Recreation and Dance
(Address above)

Dansource
P.O. Box 15038
Dallas, TX 75201
214-520-7419

Dance Teacher Now
P.O. Box 1964
West Sacramento, CA 95691
916-373-0201

Human Kinetics Publishers, Inc.
Box 5076
Champaign, IL 61825-5076

Impulse
The International Journal of Dance
Science,
Medicine, and Education
Editor: Luke Kahlich, EdD,
Available through Human
Kinetics Pub.
Box 5076
Champaign, IL 61825-5076
800-747-4457

**Kinesiology and Medicine
for Dance**
A dance journal specifically
addressing issues in health, diet,
career longevity, and training for
ballet, modern, jazz, and aerobic
dancers.
Available through Princeton
Periodicals
(See below)

The New Dance Review
c/o Anita Finkel
32 West 82nd Street, Apt. 2F
New York, NY 10024

New York On Stage
1501 Broadway, Room 2110
New York, NY 10036

**Princeton Book Company,
Publishers**
P.O. Box 57
Pennington, NJ 08534-0057
609-737-8177

Princeton Periodicals, Inc.,
a cappella books
P.O. Box 380
Pennington, NJ 08534
609-737-6525

Spotlight on Dance
Publication of the National Dance
Association/AAHPERD.
1900 Association Drive
Reston, VA 22091
703-476-3400

Stern's Performing Arts Directory
(Possibly the single best source of
information in relation to the
performing arts.)
33 West 60th Street, 10th Floor
New York, NY 10023
800-458-2845

APPENDIX E

Video Resources

A listing of where to find dance videos

Dance Film & Video Guide
(A annotated bibliography of dance films and videos.)
by Dance Films Association
Available through the Dance Book Club
12 West Delaware Avenue
Pennington, NJ 08534
800-326-7149

Hoctor Products
P.O. Box 38
Waldwick, NJ 07463
800-Hoctor-92

Kultur Video
121 Highway 36
West Long Branch, NJ 07764
201-229-2343

Jay Distributors
Box 191332
Dallas, TX 75219
800-793-6843

Cathy Roe Productions
332 Caminoe Del Monte Sol
Sante Fe, NM 87501
505-988-3597

Elektra Nonesuch/Dance Collection
75 Rockefeller Plaza
New York, NY 10019
800-222-6872

APPENDIX F

Dance Wear

Arabesque
123 North Ludlow Street
Dayton, OH 45402
800-235-6554

Art Stone
Dept. DM
1795 Express Drvie North
Smithtown, NY 11787

Ballet Barres
P.O. Box 261206
Tampa, FL 33685
800-767-1199

Baum's
106 South 11th Street
Philadelphia, PA 19108
215-923-2244

J Bloch, Inc.
818 South Broadway
9th Floor
Los Angeles, CA 90014
213-623-4227

Capezio
Ballet Makers, Inc.
Department DM1092
Totowa, NJ 07512
212-354-1887

Costume Gallery
1604 South Route 30
Burlington, NJ 08016

Curtain Call Costumes
333 East Seventh Avenue
P.O. Box 709
York, PA 17405-0709
717-852-6910

Dance Distributors
P.O. Box 11440
Harrisburg, PA 17108
800-33-Dance

The Dance Shop
2485 Forest Park Boulevard
Fort Worth, TX 76110
800-22-Dance

KD dids
P.O. Box 6119
The Bronx, NY 10451

Freed of London LTD
Dept. DMC
922 Seventh Avenue
New York, NY 10019
212-489-1055

Harlequin (Dance Floors)
3111 West Burbank Boulevard
Burbank, CA 91505
800-642-6440

Lebo's
4118 East Independence Boulevard
Charlotte, NC 28205
704-535-5000

Loshin's
260 West Mitchell Avenue
Cincinnati, OH 45232
513-541-5400

New York Dancewear Company
Discount Dancewear Catalogue
800-775-Dance

Repetto
30 Lincoln Plaza
New York, NY 10023
212-582-3900 or 800-858-5855

Jackie Sleight
4354 Laurel Canyon, #222
Studio City, CA 91604
818-763-0878

Sansha (USA), Inc.
1733 Broadway
New York, NY 10019
212-246-6212

Star Styled
P.O. Box 111805
Hialeah, FL 33011-1805

Taffy's By Mail
701 Beta Drive
Cleveland, OH 44143
216-461-3360

Weissman's Designs for Dance
1600 Macklind Avenue
St. Louis, MO 63110
314-773-9000

Wolff-Fording and Company
2220 East Main Street
Richmond, VA 23223-7503

Jazz Conventions/Competitions

(Though popular among many dance studios and students, conventions as these often represent only one view of contemporary jazz dance. Gus Giordano's annual Jazz Dance World Congress may offer a more rounded view of the art form.)

American Dance Spectrum
312 North Street
Randolph, MA 02368
617-961-Gold

Dance Caravan
P.O. Box 38
Waldwick, NJ 07463
800-Hoctor-92

Dance Educators of America
P.O. Box 509
Oceanside, NY 11572
516-766-6615

Dancefusion
P.O. Box 708
Marshall, MN 56258
507-537-7248

DanceMakers, Inc.
310 Sweetbriar Road
Greenville, SC 29615
803-244-4959

DanceMasters of America
P.O. Box 438
Independence, MO 64051-0438
816-252-0111

Dance Olympus and Danceamerica
Dept. DM
1795 Express Drive North
Smithtown, NY 11787
800-44-Dance

Dance Troupe, Inc.
P.O. Box 2326
Martinsville, VA 24113
703-956-3517

Gus Giordano
Jazz Dance Workshops and
Jazz Dance World Congress
614 Davis Street
Evanston, IL 60201
708-866-9442

I LOVE DANCE
Kim McKimmie, Director
2211 SE 76th Avenue
Portland, OR 97215
503-774-6623

L.A. Danceforce
P.O. Box 480047
Los Angeles, CA 90048
213-852-1577

Jeff Shade's Jazz Workshops
P.O. Box 4723
New York, NY 10185
212-727-9795

Regency Talent Competition
3559 Brown Road
St. Louis, MO 63114
314-429-1199

Rising Star
P.O. Box 30925
Gahanna, OH 43230
800-438-0886

Stars of Tomorrow
P.O. Box 38
Waldwick, NJ 07463
800-Hoctor-92

Tremaine Dance Conventions, Inc.
14531 Hamlin Street, #104
Van Nuys, CA 91411
818-988-8006

APPENDIX H

Preparation Checklists (Choreography)

As described in chapter 9, the most involved and time-consuming part of the creative process is the preparation phase:

- assembling the raw materials of dance;
- playing with those elements;
- using the tools of time, space, and dynamics;
- eventually formulating a "problem."

This phase requires the most research and creates the most frustration. The actual process varies considerably from choreographer to choreographer and from dance to dance. Let's look at examples of possible preparation activities and then explore one avenue of creative thought.

Assembling the Raw Materials: Music

As we emphasized in chapter 8, jazz is a music-based art, so music is a good place to begin preparation. If you hear a piece and immediately know that you want to create a dance with it, you are very lucky. Otherwise, there can be an enormous amount of research involved. Once chosen (or, as often the case in commercial choreography, once chosen for you), music can suggest a style of dance, a story, or an emotion. It can be a foil, a partner, or an enemy. Explore it ruthlessly. Insist that the music reveal all its secrets to you before you begin to put movement to beat. Following are some suggestions for music exploration using the tools of choreography, time, space, and dynamics.

Checklist: Music Exploration

Music Time

- Speed it up.
- Slow it down.
- Listen to it one whole day and one whole night.
- Move twice as fast as the music.
- Move very slowly to the music.

Music Space

- Play backwards.
- Turn down the treble.
- Turn down the bass.
- Listen to individual themes and instruments.
- Imagine the instruments are people. Where are they?
- What is the relationship of soloist to background?

Music Dynamics

- Plot the climaxes and lulls in the melody.
- Where are the surprises?
- Where is it predictable? boring?
- Do themes argue, play, or cooperate?

Once you know the music well, then just dance. Improvise (see below) with the music and without it. But don't even think of setting any steps yet. To make the dance now would be to subordinate the dance totally to the sound. You must give movement its chance to be explored as well.

Checklist: Movement Exploration (Improvisation)

It is in the preparation phase that improvisation can be used as a way of stimulating and exploring a movement idea. Improvising is allowing free rein to your movement imagination.

Time

- Begin by moving exactly to the beats in the music.
- Add beats with your body (extra steps, hip thrusts, arm movements).
- Subtract beats by moving slowly, sustaining a movement over two beats, four beats, or for an entire phrase of music.
- Make your own syncopation. Put in a body beat where it is not expected.
- Take a step (e.g., a kick-ball-change), then explore it, take it apart, repeat one part of it (kick-kick-ball-change, kick-ball-change-ball-change), do it while turning, do it backward, do it on the floor, do it in the air, do it with your arms, do it small, do it big.
- Take a combination from class and see how it fits with different music.
- Use one step you know and make it fit to this music.

Space

- See what movement ideas come from the space you are in right now.
- Dance in the aisles of the audience.
- Dance in the back of the room.
- Dance offstage and move it onstage.
- Dance lying on the floor.
- Dance in the air.
- Dance backward.
- How can you alter space?
- What about a line down the middle of the space?
- What about a picture frame off to the side?

Dynamics

- Take a step (e.g., a kick-ball-change), then:
  - kick something angrily;
  - move it hard to soft;
  - move sloppily;
  - move tenderly;
  - vary the dynamics within the phrase;
  - repeat it over and over, changing dynamics over time.

Assembling an Imaginary Creative Team

Checklist: Costumes

Costumes can have an enormous impact on the dance, altering time, space, and dynamics of movement. Costume exploration will reveal a wealth of dance ideas. Think of Fred and Ginger et al. doing the carioca in black and white costumes. Think of the mysterious alteration of character that a mask might make. Try:

- capes;
- full skirts;
- headpieces;
- gloves and spats;
- costumes that transform;
- costumes that go on and off.
- How do the costumes move, and what does that movement mean?
- What effect do colors have on movement?

Props

Fred Astaire was famous for his clever use of props as subjects for a dance. His props included a coatrack, firecrackers, his top hat and cane, sand, a revolving room, and an airplane with dancers on the wings. Today, on Broadway, Susan Stroman has inherited Astaire's fascination with props, even turning female dancers and lengths of rope into bass fiddles. She says her use of props grows out of the story line and the character. "A prop is not something plopped into a dance for clever effect. Instead, it is something that the character would naturally have."

Stroman also notes that some dancers have trouble coordinating props with the dance since they are not used to working with props in a dance class. Working with canes, hats, and costumes would be a nice adjunct to a jazz dance class.

Ideas

All dances have at their base a theme. Themes can grow from anything, any part of the dance preparation. Any of the suggestions that have been made so far are rather mechanical, but think of them as stepping-off points for theme and development. One clever prop or unusual music treatment will trigger another more important idea, which will spark something else, and that's how dances grow.

Example of a Dance

Let's pretend your jazz dance teacher has asked you to choreograph something, the only restriction being that you must use "classic jazz" music—not rap, rock and roll, or pop. You decide to use big band music from the forties. You've always liked "Boogie Woogie Bugle Boy," so you find a copy of the original recording by the Andrews Sisters. After playing it several times, it seems too slow for your taste. You speed it up a bit. The tempo is good, but the voices are too high. Try it even faster; the voices are frantic! Could be interesting. . . .

You start dancing to this frantic, shrill music. The steps come fast and furious—totally out of control. Here's an idea: a silly jitterbug with bodies flying all over the place, up and out and down: a late night at the Savoy Ballroom? No, it won't work; you don't have a partner to help you fly, and, no, this music won't work, so you look for another version and find Bette Midler's. Not exactly authentic, but it is the right tempo, and your teacher agrees to it.

So, you have some music and start to improvise. Nothing comes to mind. Your teacher shows you some steps from the forties, the Suzy Q, the Shorty George. There's one with an index finger pointing up next to the ear and wiggling while you do: step-hop on the right, then left, foot. That finger's cute, but these steps are usually done with a partner and this is a solo work.

Solo work, solo work . . . hmmm . . . so is the boogie woogie bugle boy. He's solo—at least that's what the lyrics imply. He's playing "Revele" in the morning to wake up the other soldiers. So he's alone, by himself, in the cold, before dawn. It might be interesting to contrast his loneliness with the energy and joy of the song. You might start with a very sleepy soldier dragging his bugle behind him as he crawls out of bed and drags himself to his hilltop. Hmmm. Where can you get a bugle?

Okay, here's a bugle. What can you do with it? You can pretend to blow it. You can throw and catch it, like a baton—or like the jitterbug dancers throw and catch each other. You can dance with the bugle as if it were a dancing partner! This could work. Put a wig on it and lipstick. No, that's going too far. Let's stick to the dance.

Maybe the lyrics of the song will give you an idea. Our bugle boy makes the company of soldiers "jump." Well, there are lots of "jumps" in the music—places with a sudden, sharp, unexpected beat—maybe you could catch the bugle every time the music jumps, or even jump yourself. Maybe those jumps happen in spite of your sleepiness, without you controlling them. Maybe they wake you up and get you dancing. Maybe they get the whole *company* dancing: dancers can come in from everywhere—stage right, stage left. They're dancing in the aisles, just like at the Paramount Theatre in 1938. Who? There is nobody else: this is a solo work. Maybe you can go in the aisles and get someone from the audience to dance with. No, that's too complicated and too risky. (Maybe the one you pick will have a sprained ankle.)

Back to the first idea: a lonely bugle player crawling across the stage at dawn. He gets more and more energy as the music plays, until he's really dancing happily with his bugle. What else is there about being a soldier in World War II that might give you an idea? Well, this *is* a war, and our bugle boy is not waking up his friends to go dancing; he's waking them up to kill people or possibly be killed themselves. That puts a different tone on the dance. Maybe our bugle player gets shot at the end, and the music cuts off before the end of the song. Maybe "Boogie Woogie Bugle Boy" turns into "Taps," the song traditionally played at military funerals.

This is a good idea, a late-century revisionist version of a happy, escapist, midcentury song.

But, it's hard to die onstage without getting melodramatic, and you don't really want to dance a death scene. . . . So, maybe your bugle boy is just "not there" one morning. That would mean you would have to stage the dance so that there is more than one morning, a series of mornings. That's it! Every time the chorus of the song repeats, you could start a new day, and the bugle boy gets out of bed all over again . . . except one day, when he's just not there anymore.

The music is still going, however. It has to change somehow; it has to get sadder. It can fade—get softer and softer—as the lights dim.

But you like the idea of ending with "Taps," and if the lights dim and the music fades as well, the audience will think the dance is over and start to applaud . . . hopefully. How about this: as the stage lights start to dim, a single spot comes up somewhere else. Where? At the back of the audience, or on the side, or in a window. And there is a lonely dancer in black, playing . . . or dancing . . . to "Taps."

So here we are at the end of the preparation phrase. You have an idea, a problem formulated. That a very good place to start. You also have a potential beginning, middle, and an end, but it is all theoretical—the dance equivalent of a first draft. Who knows what it will be like when it's finished, after incubation, illumination, and polishing, when it's moving, when it's a dance.

(NOTE: Though this study is in no way similar to his dance, the death theme was suggested by Paul Taylor's masterpiece "Company B" in which dying soldiers are contrasted with happy young couples dancing to the music of the Andrews Sisters.)

Some Last Words of Advice

- Try not to take anything to seriously.
- Don't accept the first idea that comes to you just because you're so happy to have an idea.
- Keep exploring.

- Keep playing.
- The good ideas will stick.

This is not an easy process. Learning to choreograph is learning to create something out of anything. To a creative artist beginning a new work, every force in the universe (for example, space, time, dynamics, motion, thought, and imagination) is available, and nothing is so frightening to man as freedom. But reassuringly, choreography is a skill and, as we've tried to do here, it can be broken down into stages (even if the stages don't necessarily follow one another). From those stages that reverse and retreat and encircle and go back then forth, a dance can be forged and enriched until it becomes a work of art.

Jazz Timeline

When	Jazz/Popular Music	Composers/Performers	Popular and Stage Dance	Choreographers/Performers	Tunes/Shows
Pre-20th Century	Folk music Spirituals Brass band music Medicine shows-Eccentric dancing Buddy Bolden Band plays New Orleans streets (1894) Blues, minstrels show—(secular) Gospel—religious Creole synthesis Ragtime	Bert Williams, George Walker (Juba) Eubie Blake/piano (Baltimore) Scott Joplin rags are published New Orleans march music Midwest	Minstrel shows (1830s) Call and Response, Ring Shouts The Cakewalk, the Buzzard Lope, Juba and Patting Juba, Voodoo (Shoulders), Calinda, Congo (antecedent of Twist) The Shuffle, Patting, the Slow Drag, The waltz, polka, masurka, quadrille	Maire Bonfanti	The Black Crook (1866) Maple Leaf Rag (1899) Chocolate Creams Cakewalk (1901) Vaudeville (1890–1920)
1900	Popular music was based on what was popular in Europe Bluegrass—(blues and Irish jigs) Jazz activity centered in New Orleans	European-American Southern whites Jelly Roll Morton New Orleans (1902) Buddy Bolden King Oliver	The Buzzard Lope The Cakewalk from the days of the slaves National dance crazes: The Funky Butt, the Slow Drag, Eagle Rock, Shimmy, Grind, the Itch Buck & Wing (clog & jig with syncopated rhythms) "Walkin' the Dog," (dance songs with instructions) Precision dance, The Castlewalk, the Gavotte	The Whitman Sisters George M. Cohan Maxie McCree	Bill Bailey (1902) Scott Joplin's ragtime opera A Guest of Honor (1903) National Ragtime Contest (1904) St. Louis Rag (1903) Little Johnny Jones (1904) Alexander's Ragtime Band (1911) S. Joplin opera: Treemonisha (1911)
1910s	Jim Crow laws close down Storyville in New Orleans "Blues" comes into general use as a musical term Ragtime—Alexander's Ragtime Band (1911) Ballads (1914)	King Oliver & W.C. Handy Louis Armstrong moves to Chicago Irving Berlin (1888–1989) Jerome Kern (1885–1945)		Ned Wayburn—dance director Irene & Vernon Castle	Ziegfeld Follies (1914) Watch Your Step Yip Yip Yaphunk (Berlin)

When	Jazz/Popular Music	Composers/Performers	Popular and Stage Dance	Choreographers/Performers	Tunes/Shows
1920s	Big bands begin (1916) First band that stressed written arrangements Boogie-woogie recorded (Pinetop Smith 1928)	James P. Johnson slide piano concerto (1921) Fletcher Henderson Bix Beiderbecke Duke Ellington opens at the Cotton Club (1927) Sidney Bechet goes to Paris (1928) Paul Whiteman	Black Bottom Dance specialities The Charleston Eccentric dancing, acrobatics, soft-shoe The height, then the wane, of tap dance Buck and Wing	Adalaide & Hughes/ Ray Bolger Johnny Nit/Eddie Rector Ethel Waters Josephine Baker Bill Robinson Seymour Felix	*Shuffle Along* (1921) *Poor Little Ritz Girl* (1920) *Runnin' Wild* (1923) *Rhapsody in Blue* (1924) *Lady Be Good* (1925) Gershwin *Liza, Dixie to Broadway* *Peggy Ann* (1926) Rodgers & Hart *Showboat* (1927) Hammerstein & Kern
1930s	White version, concert vs. dance band The Cotton Club 52nd Street (Swing St.) at height Orchestrated boogie-woogie, swing Kansas City blues Count Basie discovered 1935 Featured singers in big bands Great pianists Benny Goodman becomes the first big white star of jazz using Fletcher Henderson arrangements Count Basie Louis Jordan combo Benny Goodman at Carnegie Hall (1938)	Fats Waller Dorsey Brothers Duke Ellington/ Louis Armstrong Benny Goodman, w/ Gene Krupa and Harry James, succeeds in Calif. (1935) Billie Holiday and Joe Williams Cole Porter (1891–1964) Fats Waller & Art Tatum Schwartz & Dietz Irving Berlin, Rodgers and Hart Ira & George Gershwin Benny Goodman Artie Shaw, Glenn Miller Jimmy & Tommy Dorsey	Gershwin & Broadway The Hoofers Club was headquarters for American tap dance from now through the forties Dance coordinated with the book of the show The Savoy Ballroom, where the great musicians inspired the great dancers and vice versa for 30 years Dance became the Lindy-Hop, Jitterbug Ballroom influence, ballet, and tap Ballet influence Integration of plot and choreography	Busby Berkeley Buddy Bradley (Choreographer for musicals and ballet in Europe) Nicholas Brothers (through '50s) Fred & Adele Astaire Robert Alton— Fred Astaire/Hermes Pan George Balanchine Jerome Robbins Agnes DeMille	*42nd Street* (1933), *Dames* (1934), *Gold Diggers* of '33, '35, '37 *Girl Crazy* ('30), *Porgy & Bess* ('35) Gershwin *Sun Valley Serenade* *The Big Broadcast* ('41) *The Band Wagon* ('31) Rasch *Pal Joey* ('40) *Anything Goes* ('34) Porter *Flying Down to Rio* ('33) *Top Hat* ('36), *On Your Toes* ('36) Balanchine

When	Jazz/Popular Music	Composers/Performers	Popular and Stage Dance	Choreographers/Performers	Tunes/Shows
1940s			Begin shift from amateur vernacular to professional jazz: vernacular + modern and ballet Afro-Haitian influence	Pearl Primus, Katherine Dunham Bobby Van Jack Cole/Marge & Gower Champion	*Oklahoma* ('43) *Stormy Weather* ('43) *Fancy Free* ('44) *On the Town* ('45) *Carousel* ('45) DeMille
Late 1940s	Be bop Jazz becomes more music for listening Combined jazz and *Afro-Cuban* music The Latin invasion Big bands begin to fade out	Charlie Parker Bud Powell Dizzy Gillespie Lerner & Loewe	Jazz influenced by modern dance Orient, Latin America, and Harlem influence Isolations and flow Latin invasion, the Mambo, the Cha Cha	Hanya Holm on Broadway	*Kiss Me Kate* ('48), *South Pacific* ('49),
1950s	Electric guitar bass Rhythm and blues Electric boogie-woogie takes over as new dance music R & B becomes Rock & Roll Cool jazz—Hard bop	Frank Loesser (1910–1969) Richard Adler and Jerry Ross Charles Brown, Ruth Brown, Fats Domino Mahalia Jackson at Carnegie Hall Sondheim & Bernstein Jules Styne & Stephen Sondheim Chuck Berry/The Cadillacs Miles Davis, Stan Getz, and Gil Evans, Art Blakely, Sonny Rollins, Clifford Brown	The Mambo Begin era of director-choreographer Blending dancing, drama, and decor Locomotion, Mashed Potato, Fly Jazz dance and music begin to separate	Hermes Pan Gene Kelly Bob Fosse/Gwen Verdon Donald MacKayle Jerome Robbins Talley Beatty Carol Haney Alvin Ailey, Donald Byrd Cholly Atkins for pop performers Debbie Reynolds, Peter Gennaro Michael Kidd, Luigi, Matt Mattox, Gower Champion	*Guys & Dolls* ('50) *Showboat* ('51) *An American in Paris* ('51) Robbins *Kismet* ('53) Cole *Small-town Girl* ('53) *Can-Can* ('53) *Singin' in the Rain* ('53) Champion *Pajama Game* ('54) Fosse *Three for the Show* ('55) *Damn Yankees* ('55) *My Fair Lady* ('56) *West Side Story* ('57) *Flower Drum Song* ('58) *Blues Suite* ('58) *Gypsy* ('59) Robbins American Bandstand (Through '80s)

When	Jazz/Popular Music	Composers/Performers	Popular and Stage Dance	Choreographers/Performers	Tunes/Shows
1960s	English invasion The Beatles had listened to great blues artists as well as rock & roll	Leadbelly, Muddy Waters Howlin Wolf, Sonny Terry Brownie McGhee	TV the medium of the moment for dance		Bye Bye Birdie ('60) Movie version: West Side Story ('60) Carnival ('61) The Unsinkable Molly Brown ('64)
	Brazilian invasion—bossa nova, samba Soul music, Motown Avant-garde jazz Electric jazz, fusion	Stan Getz Aretha Franklin/Supremes Ornette Coleman Miles Davis	Twist, Pony, Hully Gully, Boogaloo, Watusi	Gus Giordano Jerome Robbins: Export	Seven Brides for Seven Brothers Hello Dolly ('64) TV variety shows/specials Fiddler on the Roof ('64) Sweet Charity ('67) Opus Jazz
1970s	Computerized drum beat Deejays Most pop music will be completely computerized except for the singer by 1985 Influence of salsa nd reggae		Brassy, accelerated pace of urban life reflected ultra-professional, exhibitionism, sensuality Movement with psych insight of character The Hustle, disco dancing	Jaime Rogers Bob Fosse Michael Bennett John Travolta Tremaine, Simonson Kenny Ortega Tommy Tune	Pippin ('72) Fosse Cabaret ('73) Chicago ('75) Fosse A Chorus Line ('75) Saturday Night Fever ('77) Dancin' ('78) All That Jazz ('79) Fosse
1980s	Music videos Rap emerges	Young Lions: Wynton Marsalis, et. al. Andrew Lloyd Weber	Enter MTV, editing effects onstaging dance Break dancing Social forms: Hip-hop, aerobic dancing Repetitive, gross motor movements Vogueing, Lyrical jazz is back	Michael Jackson Michael Peters Hammer Paula Abdul Instilling old forms with new feeling Nostalgia	Revival of 42nd Street ('80) Champion Cats ('82) Nine ('82) My One and Only ('83) Flashdance ('83) Thriller ('84) video A Chorus Line ('85), the movie, by R. Attenborough

When	Jazz/Popular Music	Composers/ Performers	Popular and Stage Dance	Choreographers/ Performers	Tunes/ Shows
1990s			Revivals		
	Jazz and rap mix	Frank Loesser (Composer) 1992 Rivival *Guys and Dolls/The Most Happy Fella*		Christopher Chadman	*Jerome Robbins'* Broadway ('90) *Grant Hotel* ('90) Tune *Guys and Dolls* (Orig. 1942, Rev. 1992) Rev. 1992
		Miles Davis (postmortem) with guests	Music videos/Techno-hop	Hope Clark Gregory Hines Susan Stroman Jamal Graves Vincent Paterson	*Jelly's Last Jam* ('92) *Crazy for You* ('92) Madonna and Michael Jackson videos (1988–1989)
				Rosie Perez	In Living Color's Fly Girls
			Rave	Wayne Cilento	*Tommy* (on Broadway) ('93)

APPENDIX J

Suggested Reading

Alexander, F.M. *Constructive Conscious Control of the Individual.* London: Methuen and Co., 1924.

_____. *The Use of the Self.* New York: E.P. Dutton & Co., Inc., Publishers, 1932.

Alter, J. *Stretch and Strengthen.* Boston: Houghton Mifflin Co., 1986.

_____. *Surviving Exercise.* Boston: Houghton Mifflin Co., 1983.

Arnheim, D. *Dance Injuries: Their Prevention and Care.* Princeton: Princeton Book Company, Publishers, 1986.

Astaire, Fred. *Steps in Time.* New York: Harper and Row, 1959.

Audy, Robert. *Tap Dancing.* New York: Vintage, 1976.

Baral, Robert. *Revue: The Great Broadway Period.* New York: Fleet Press, 1970.

Barron, Frank. *Artists in the Making.* New York: Seminar Press, 1972. (especially chpt. 8 by J. Alter on Dancers)

Bartinieff, I., and D. Lewis. *Body Movement: Coping With the Environment.* New York: Gordon and Breach Science Publishers, 1980.

Barardi, G. *Finding Balance.* New Jersey: Dance Horizons, Princeton Book Company, Publishers, 1991.

Bernstein, Leonard. *The Joy of Music.* New York: Simon and Shuster, 1959.

Bordman, Gerald. *The American Musical Theatre.* New York: Oxford University Press, 1982.

California State Department of Education, Visual and Performing Arts Framework and Criteria Committee. *Visual and Performing Arts Framework for California Public Schools: K through Grade 12.* Janet Lundin and Theodore Smith, eds. Sacramento, Calif.: 1982.

Castle, Irene. *Castles in the Air.* New York: DaCapo Press, 1980.

Cayou, Dolores. *Modern Jazz Dance.* London: Dance Books Ltd., 1976.

Chmelar, R., and S. Fitt. *Diet: A Complete Guide to Nutrition and Weight Control.* Princeton: Princeton Book Company, Publishers, 1990.

Clark, N. *Sports Nutrition Guidebook: Eating to Fuel Your Active Lifestyle.* Champaign, Ill.: Leisure Press, 1990.

Croce, Arlene. *The Fred Astaire and Ginger Rogers Book.* New York: Dutton, 1972.

Davis, G.A. *Creativity is Forever,* 2nd ed. Dubuque: Kendall Hunt Publishing Company, 1983.

DeMille, Agnes. *America Dances.* New York: Macmillan, 1980.

DeMille, Agnes. *Dance to the Piper/And Promenade Home.* New York: DaCapo, 1980.

Dissanayake, Ellen. *What Is Art For?* Seattle, Wash.: University of Washington Press, 1988.

——————. *Homo Aestheticus.* New York: The Free Press, 1992.

Dow, A., and M. Michaelson. *The Official guide to Jazz Dancing.* Secaucus, N.J.: Chartwell Books, Inc., 1980.

Draper, Paul. *Paul Draper on Tap Dancing.* New York: M. Dekker, 1978.

DuBois, W.E.B. *The Souls of Black Folk.* Chicago: A.C. McLurge and Company, 1903.

Dunham, Katherine. *Island Possessed.* Garden City, N.Y.: Doubleday, 1969.

Ellington, Duke. *Music is My Mistress.* Garden City, N.Y.: Doubleday, 1973.

Emery, Lynne Fauley. *Black Dance in the United States from 1619 to Today.* 2d rev. ed. Pennington, N.J.: Princeton Book Co., 1988.

Fitt, S. *Dance Kinesiology.* New York: Schirmer Books, 1988.

Fox, Paula. *Slave Dancer.* New York: Dell Publishing Company, 1973.

Frich, Elisabeth. *The Matt Mattox Book of Jazz Dance.* New York: Sterling, 1983.

Gardner, Howard. *Art, Mind and Brain.* New York: Basic Books, 1982.

——————. *The Arts and Human Development: A Psychology Study of the Artistic Process.* New York: Wiley, 1973.

——————. *Frames of Mind: The Theory of Multiple Intelligences.* New York: Basic Books, Inc., Publishers, 1985.

Gelb, M. *Body Learning: An Introduction to the Alexander Technique.* New York: G.P. Putnam & Sons, 1980.

Getzels, J., and Mihalyi Csikszentmihalyi. *The Creative Vision: A Longitudinal Study of Problem-Finding in Art.* New York: Wiley-Interscience, 1976.

Gillespie, Dizzy with Al Fraser, *To Be, or Not . . . to Bop.* Garden City, N.Y.: Doubleday, 1979.

Gottfried, Martin. *All His Jazz: The Life and Death of Bob Fosse.* New York: Bantam, 1990.

——————. *Broadway Musicals.* New York: Abrams, 1984.

Grant, G. *Technical Manual and Dictionary of Classical Ballet.* New York: Dover Publications, 1970.

Gregory, J. *Understanding Ballet.* London: Octopus Books Limited, 1972.

Haskins, Jim. *The Cotton Club.* New York: Random House Inc. of New York, 1977.

Hirshorn, Clive. *The Hollywood Musical.* New York: Crown, 1981.

Huggins, Nathan Irvin. *Harlem Renaissance.* New York: Oxford University Press, Inc., 1971.

Humphrey, Doris. *The Art of Making Dances.* Pennington, N.J.: Princeton Book Co., 1987.

Isaacs, B., and J. Kobler. *The Nickolaus Technique.* New York: A & W Visual Library, 1978.

Jackson, Irene, ed. *More than Dancing: Essays on Afro-American Music and Musicians.* Westport, Conn.: Greenwood Press, 1985.

Jones, F.P. *Body Awareness in Action.* New York: Schocken Books, 1976.

Jones, LeRoi. *Black Music.* New York: William Morrow, 1968.

Kimball, Robert, and William Bolcom. *Reminiscing with Sissle and Blake.* New York: The Viking Press, 1973.

Kirkland, Gelsey, with Greg Lawrence. *Dancing on My Grave.* New York: Doubleday, 1986.

Kislan, Richard. *Hoofing on Broadway: A History of Show Dancing.* New York: Prentice-Hall Press, 1987.

Kleinman, M. *The Acquisition of Motor Skill.* Princeton: Princeton Book Company, Publishers, 1983.

Kohut, D. *Musical Performance Learning Theory and Pedagogy.* Englewood Cliffs, N.J.: Prentice-Hall, Inc., 1985.

Kraus, R., Chapman, S. and B. Dixon. *History of the Dance in Art and Education,* 3rd ed. Englewood Cliffs, N.J.: Prentice-Hall, Inc., 1991.

Lamb, W., and E. Watson. *Body Code: The Meaning in Movement.* Princeton: Princeton Book Company, Publishers, 1987.

Leibowitz, J, and B. Connington. *The Alexander Technique.* New York: Harper & Row, Publishers, 1990.

Lewis, D. *The Illustrated Dance Technique of Jose Limon.* New York: Harper & Row, Publishers, 1984.

Loney, Glenn, ed. *Musical Theatre in America.* Westport, Conn.: Greenwood Press, 1981.

_____. *Unsung Genius: The Passion of Dancer-Choreographer Jack Cole.* New York: Franklin Watts, 1984.

Luigi, and Kenneth Wydro. *The Luigi Jazz Dance Technique.* Garden City, N.Y.: Doubleday, 1981.

Mandelbaum, Ken. *A Chorus Line and the Musicals of Michael Bennett.* New York: St. Martins Press, 1975.

Mates, Julian. *America's Musical Stage: Two Hundred Years of Musical Theatre.* Westport, Conn.: Greenwood Press, 1985.

May, Rollo. *The Courage to Create.* New York: W.W. Norton, 1975.

McCabe, John. *George M. Cohan: The Man Who Owned Broadway.* Garden City, N.Y.: Doubleday and Co., 1973.

Moshe, F. *Awareness Through Movement.* New York: Harper and Row, 1972.

Mueller, John. *Astaire Dancing.* New York: Alfred A. Knopf, 1984.

Murray, Albert. *Stomping the Blues.* New York: McGraw-Hill, 1976.

Nagrin, D. *How to Dance Forever: Surviving Against the Odds.* New York: William Morrow and Co., Inc., 1988.

Olsen, A. *Body Stories: A Guide to Experiential Anatomy.* Barrytown, New York: Staton Hill Press, 1991.

Paskevska, A. *Ballet: From the First Plié to Mastery.* Princeton: Dance Horizons/Princeton Book Company, Publishers, 1990.

Philip, F., and E. Gail *The Pilates Method of Physical and Mental Conditioning.* New York: Warner Books, 1980.

Rothenberg, A. and C. R. Hausman, eds. *The Creativity Question.* Durham, N.C.: Duke University Press, 1976.

Sampson, Henry T. *Blacks in Blackface: A Source Book on Early Black Musical Shows.* Metuchen, N.J.: Scarecrow Press Inc., 1980.

Sobel, Machel. *Travelin' On: The Slave Journey to an Afro-Baptist Faith.* Westport, Conn.: Greenwood Press, 1979.

Sterns, Marshall, and Jean Stearns. *Jazz Dance: The Story of American Vernacular Dance.* New York: Macmillan and Co., 1968.

Schirmer, 1968.

Stodelle, E. *The Dance Technique of Doris Humphrey and Its Creative Potential.* Princeton, N.J.: Dance Horizons/Princeton Book Company, Publishers, 1978.

Thomas, Tony. *That's Dancing.* New York: Abrams, 1984.

———. *The Films of Gene Kelly: Song and Dance Man.* Secaucus, N.J.: Citadel Press, 1974.

———, and Jim Terry with Busby Berkeley. *The Busby Berkeley Book.* Greenwich, Conn.: New York Graphic Society, 1973.

Todd, M. *The Thinking Body.* Princeton, N.J.: A Dance Horizons Book/Princeton Book Company, Publishers, 1968.

Toll, Robert C. *On with the Show, The First Century of Show Business in America.* New York: Oxford University Press, 1976.

Traguth, Fred. *Modern Jazz Dance.* Englewood Cliffs, N.J.: Prentice-Hall, 1983.

Wallace, Graham. *In the Creativity Question.* edited by Albert Rothenberg and Carl R. Hausman. Durham, N.C.: Duke University Press, 1976.

Warren, G. W. *Classical Ballet Technique.* Tampa: University of F.L. Press, 1989.

Watkins, A, and P. Clarkson. *Dancing Longer, Dancing Stronger: A Dancer's Guide to Improving Technique and Preventing injury.* Princeton: Dance Horizons/Princeton Book Company, Publishers, 1990.

Wayburn, Ned. *The Art of Stage Dancing.* New York: Ned Wayburn Studios, 1925.

Williams, J. M., ed. *Applied Sports Psychology: Personal Growth to Peak Performance.* Mountain View: Mayfield Publishing Co., 1986.

Winner, Ellen. *Invented Worlds: The Psychology of the Arts.* Cambridge, Mass.: Harvard University Press, 1982.

Winearls, Jane. *Choreography: The Art of the Body.* London: Dance Books, 1990.

Periodicals

Kerr, Walter. "Eubie!" *New York Times,* 22 September 1978.

Kroll, Jack. "A Buck, A Wing and a Smile." *Newsweek,* 9 January 1984.

Maultsby, Portia K. "West African Influences in U.S. Black Music." *Western Journal of Black Studies* (Pullman, Wash.: Black Studies Program/ Washington State University Press) vol. 3, no. 3 (Fall 1979): 197–215.

Minns, Al, and Leon James. "Popular Dances from the Cakewalk to Watusi." *Ebony,* August 1961.

Ostiere, Beryl Hilary. "Susan Stroman's Dream Season." *Dance Magazine,* May 1992, 36–37.

Prevots, Naima. "Dancing in the Sun: Hollywood Choreographers." Ph.D. diss., Ann Arbor, Mich.: University Microfilms, 1987.

Smith, N. Weight Control in the Athlete. *Clinics in Sports Medicine,* Vol. 3:3:693, 1984.

Winter, Marian Hannah. "Juba and American Minstrelsy." *Dance Index,* February 1947, 28–48.

MODELS

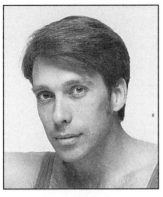

Joseph Doucette
Joey Doucette, dancer and choreographer, has performed with many Latin American stars. He has lived and worked in Mexico City, New York, and Los Angeles. He recently finished a show for Trump's Taj Mahal in Atlantic City and is currently working on a show starring Olga Breeskin at the Normandie Casino in Los Angeles.

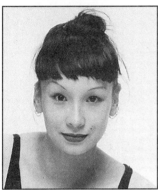

Johanna Lynne
Johanna Lynne studied ballet with the Princeton Ballet and the Joffrey Ballet. She has been awarded scholarships for the Hubbard Street Theatre, Alvin Ailey, and Steps in New York. She is currently working in regional theatre and industrial shows and would like to dance on Broadway.

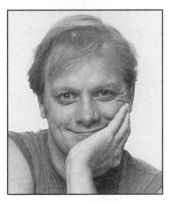

Francis Roach
Francis Roach, dancer and choreographer, performs on television and in films in New York, where his performance credits include appearances with Liza Minnelli, Shirley MacLaine, Gene Kelly, and the Pointer Sisters. Roach, protégé of jazz dance legend Luigi, has also performed and taught in Japan, Italy, South Africa, Brazil, and Puerto Rico.

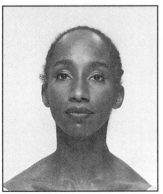

Cheryl Whitney-Marcuard
Cheryl Whitney-Marcuard received a B.A. in English literature and Music from St. Lawrence University. She began her dance training at Peabody Conservatory and received an M.S. in ballet from Indiana University. She has performed with companies in the Washington D.C. region. She currently teaches in Princeton, NJ at the Center for Music and Young Children, Aparri Ballet, and the Princeton Ballet School. Her other teaching credits include the New Jersey Governor's School for the Arts, Peabody Conservatory, Baltimore School for the Arts, Howard University, and Indiana University.

INDEX